Yoga for Beginners

Basic Yoga Poses for Flexibility, Stress Relief, and Inner Peace

(Guided Meditations for Deep Relaxation, Healing Sleep, and Quieting the Mind)

Rolf Swanson

Published by Rob Miles

Rolf Swanson

All Rights Reserved

Yoga for Beginners: Basic Yoga Poses for Flexibility, Stress Relief, and Inner Peace (Guided Meditations for Deep Relaxation, Healing Sleep, and Quieting the Mind)

ISBN 978-1-989990-57-5

Legal & Disclaimer

The information contained in this book is not designed to replace or take the place of any form of medicine or professional medical advice. The information in this book has been provided for educational and entertainment purposes only.

The information contained in this book has been compiled from sources deemed reliable, and it is accurate to the best of the Author's knowledge; however, the Author cannot guarantee its accuracy and validity and cannot be held liable for any errors or omissions. Changes are periodically made to this book. You must consult your doctor or get professional medical advice before using any of the suggested remedies, techniques, or information in this book.

Table of Contents

INTRODUCTION...1

CHAPTER 1:THE BENEFITS OF YOGA 4

CHAPTER 2: THE FUNDAMENTALS OF NIYAMA...............20

CHAPTER 3: HEALING YOUR BODY WITH YOGA...............29

CHAPTER 4: FIVE FINGERS FOR FIVE ELEMENTS...............34

CHAPTER 5: SIMPLE AND BASIC YOGA POSES.................39

CHAPTER 6: YOGA POSES FOR WEIGHT LOSS..................47

CHAPTER 7: BREATHING TECHNIQUES...........................58

CHAPTER 8: HIP RELIEF 68

CHAPTER 9: POSES FOR MIND CLARITY AND FOCUS........88

CHAPTER 10: BREATHER EXERCISES AND MEDITATION ...99

CHAPTER 11: WEIGHT LOSS..107

CHAPTER 12: EXTENDED TRIANGLE POSE 115

CHAPTER 13: SOME IMPORTANT BREATHING EXERCISES
TO PRACTICE AT HOME 123

CHAPTER 14: YOGA AND WEIGHT LOSS.........................146

CHAPTER 15: THE FORWARD BENDS 151

CHAPTER 16: HOT YOGA..155

CHAPTER 17: YOGA EXERCISES FOR BEGINNERS...........164

CHAPTER 18: PRANAYAMA – WEIGHT LOSS BREATHING EXERCISES 170

CHAPTER 19: THE KOAN OF YOGA 181

CONCLUSION 192

Yoga for beginners is now super easy to learn. For those who have never attended any yoga programs before, it does not matter. Within the course of yoga for beginners, The Yogis (the person who practices yoga and contains realized a higher amount of psychic perception) focuses on the marriage of head, body and nature and declares that this is attained during the yoga practices and techniques. The Yogis believes that one's mind and body were strapped into a good design. If this is the first time you've read about yoga, you will certainly marvel on how yoga exercises are done and just how it seems. You will also know which type of yoga position is going to be best for you.

Yoga has conducted a remarkable procedure of healing someone through equilibrium. Yoga may be properly performed when you are in the right environment. With the awesome effects of yoga, several doctors have already been convinced that this exercise also gives therapeutic benefits, plus they can recommend this exercise for those who have hard to cure illnesses. Try to study the roles of yoga if you have suffered from a long time disease.

You must first genuinely believe that this exercise will help you be restored or to become cured before exercising the positions of yoga. The opportunities of yoga are extremely exciting to execute. As a novice, you'll find it not too difficult to carry on using the workouts because it is very simple. The yoga process adds movement that is great for your body organs and it also involves moving parts of your body which are rarely stimulated. Some simple rules of yoga for novices are actually similar to those who are already practicing yoga; they include the standing poses, the seated poses, ahead and backward stability together with bends and twisting. The intense poses and opportunities will be handled in the latter part of the yoga exercise. You can discover the opportunities of yoga for newbies at home or any yoga course. However, as you are a starter, the main thing you need to know is your self-control. It is not merely about performing yoga since it does not matter whether it's yoga for newbies or yoga for the master.

CHAPTER 1: THE BENEFITS OF YOGA

The practice of yoga has gone through a lot of changes through time. It has adapted to the needs of its practitioners and those who are interested to learn more about it. One thing remains the same despite the changes – the goal, and that is to unite the inner and outer qualities of life.

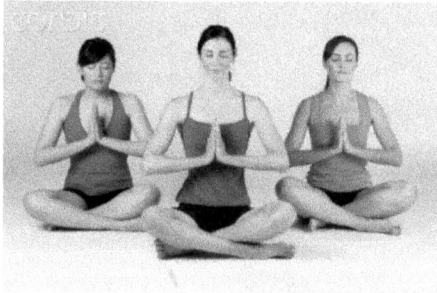

Yoga is sometimes performed in certain religious practices, but this is not a religious system. It is mainly taught as a system of exercises and physical poses that are targeted to improve your health and general well-being. There is more to yoga than what is being taught. You can further indulge in its complex ideas if you are serious in learning more about the matter on a deeper level.

Yoga involves different techniques, poses and practices that are all aimed at helping you to become one with the universe. This can be achieved by unifying your mind, body and spirit until you get to the state of enlightenment. It comes in many forms, which gives out a lot of benefits that include the following:

1. Better body posture

Poor posture can have many ill effects on your health, which include problems with your neck, joints, back and muscles. If you allow your body to slump, this will affect your neck and lower back, which can lead to degenerative arthritis of the spine.

2. Improved flexibility

You will notice the big difference with how your body is able to follow even the most difficult yoga poses as you continue with the practice. Do not force yourself to perfect the yoga poses on your first try. Reach as far as you can, but stop when you start feeling pains.

3. Stronger muscles

Strong muscles do not only make you look good, they also protect you from conditions, such as back pain and arthritis.

4. Stronger bones

You will learn how to lift your own weight as you practice more yoga poses. This will protect you from developing osteoporosis. The practice also lowers the levels of your stress hormone that is known as cortisol. As a result, the calcium in the bones remains intact, which makes the bones healthier and stronger.

5. Healthier lifestyle

Yoga is a form of exercise and it helps you burn calories with the movements that are involved. It also addresses your emotional and spiritual being. What seems to be a simple weight problem may be more complex than how you perceive it to be. This may already be rooted to certain emotional baggage that the practice will help you to understand and address.

6. Protects your spine

A well-balanced asana practice will result to spinal discs that are more flexible because it requires you to perform a lot of twists, forward and back bends.

7. Boosts your blood flow

Aside from boosting the blood flow, yoga also helps in getting more oxygen into your system. It decreases your risks of suffering from heart attack and stroke.

8. Regular heart rate

Aside from decreasing your chances of having a heart attack, it also protects you from depression. Constant yoga practice will result to a lower resting heart rate and it will also boost your endurance. Yoga also helps in keeping your blood pressure normal.

9. Higher level of good cholesterol

Yoga increases the level of your body's good cholesterol or HDL and lowers your bad cholesterol or LDL. It also lowers your blood sugar level, which is the reason why a lot of diabetics have found an ally in this form of meditation and exercise.

10. Lower cortisol levels

Too much cortisol in the system can lead to health problems, such as insulin resistance, osteoporosis, high blood pressure and depression. It also prompts you to go on a food-seeking behavior, which means that you seek food for comfort in order to deal with whatever you are feeling. This can lead to weight gain that can worsen your health and emotional concerns.

11. Helps you stay focused

A big part of the practice involves concentration. This is not easy to achieve, especially for beginners who are used in a noise-filled environment. Yoga encourages you to seek peace and perform the exercises in silence. It teaches you how to focus and stay focused during the exercise. You can apply what you have learned in your daily activities and through time, you will see how much you've changed since you started doing yoga.

12. Relaxing

It encourages you to relax, relieves yourself from any negative vibes and helps you to focus on the present.

13. Prevents any cartilage and joint injuries

The movements that are involved in the practice push your joints to perform in a full range motion. You tend to perform less physical activities as you get older. Yoga helps your bones and joints to remain strong and become less prone to injuries.

14. Improved balance

Your proprioception increases when you make yoga a part of your lifestyle. It refers to your ability to feel where in space is your physical body and what is it doing. Having a poor proprioception is often related to old age, back pain and knee problems. It is normal for beginners to feel wobbly in performing the steps, but as your body gets used to the movements, you will have a better balance.

15. Learning how to release the tension in your limbs

There are certain habits and mannerisms that lead to chronic tension and muscle fatigue. They include the facial expressions that you often do when you are staring at your computer screen; how you grip the steering wheel with force when you are driving or hold the receiver of the phone too tight when you are talking to someone.

You begin to develop these habits unconsciously and you will only become aware of the problem once you feel soreness and pain. As you get used to yoga movements, you will eventually learn how to hold the tension from the different parts of your body. Instead of using too much force even when not needed, you will learn how to control and relax your muscles.

16. Promotes better sleep

There are certain kinds of yoga that are aimed to help you improve your sleeping patterns. This is done by giving you a better coping mechanism with your everyday struggle with life. The practices involve the downtime of your nervous system, which also make you feel less stressed and fatigued. To get these benefits, the yoga practices that you can try include yoga nidra, restorative asana, pranayama, meditation and Savasana.

They all turn your senses inward and in effect, will make you feel more relaxed.

17. Stronger immune system

Various yoga poses will require you to contract and stretch your muscles. By doing this often, there will be an increase in the drainage of lymph. As a result, your lymphatic system is able to fight infections, get rid of your body's toxins and fight off cancerous cells.

For stronger immunity, you can perform either pranayama or asana, but you can get more of this kind of benefit from doing meditation. The latter supports the immune system and boosts it whenever necessary and lowers it, if needed.

18. Healthy and easy breathing

Yoga involves lots of breathing exercises. This is actually the first thing that you will learn upon following the practice. Yoga is now being recommended to people who have lung problems. The practice follows a technique that is called complete breathing, which is specifically helpful to those who are suffering from lung problems due to congestive heart failure. As you continue with the practice, the oxygen saturation in your blood will increase. This will make it easier for you to breathe in and exhale through your nose.

19. Better you

The most important benefit of this practice is that it encourages you to believe. As the days go by, you will have more confidence and self-esteem. You will find the right ways to turn any negative thoughts into something positive. It will be easier to believe that you can do whatever you wish to do. In effect, this will push yourself to try your best and become better in everything that you do.

Yoga and Stress

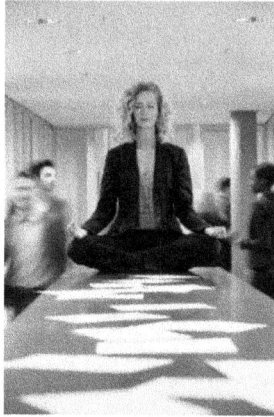

Everybody gets stressed out, no matter how old or young you are or what kind of life you have. It is bound to happen. While mild anxiety is common, it becomes a problem when it happens all the time and it begins to develop into something chronic. It is physically and emotionally draining. This can lead to worse health conditions if you will not learn how to manage and cope with stress.

The body tends to suffer more from stress if you don't exercise. This will result to tensions in the muscles and joints, difficulty in breathing and disturbed thoughts. Without realizing it, you are causing the problem to become worse than how it actually was. Through yoga practice, you will learn how to manage stress by accessing your inner strength.

You can begin by practicing daily yoga exercises, meditation and breathing techniques. As you go about it, you will learn how to regulate your breathing. This will also teach you how to relax your body by releasing muscle tensions and flushing your whole system, including your brain, with oxygen, fresh blood and essential nutrients. There are whole body exercises that you can perform, such as the Sun Poses that will teach you how to breathe deeply and steadily.

Daily yoga practice will help in training your mind to calm down whenever you are feeling overwhelmed. With the help of meditation, you are able to tap your inner resources, which make you happier and more fulfilled. In this state, you will become healthier and less dependent on medications.

Yoga brings a greater self-awareness to those who practice it on a regular basis. This is the reason why it is essential not only in relieving stress, but it also teaches you how to enjoy an everlasting physical and emotional health.

Yoga is a mind and body practice. It brings together mental and physical disciplines that help in finding peace in your body and mind. It comes in many forms, styles and complexities. There are people who choose the kinds of yoga that they will perform based on the intensity of movements, while others choose based on the benefits that they will get from the exercise.

For example, a popular style of yoga that is effective in managing stress is known as the Hatha yoga. This is common and is actually recommended for beginners because of the easy movements and slower pace. You can try the more complicated styles once you get the hang of things. The most important factor here is that you have to begin with something.

There are three core components of yoga – poses, breathing and meditation.

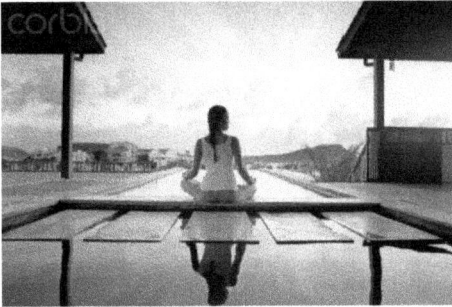

Yoga poses or postures are composed of a series of movements that are intended to make you stronger and increase your flexibility. The poses may begin with simple stretches and end with more difficult and challenging types that will test your physical limitations.

The practice will teach you how to control your breathing. Through this, you will also learn how to control your body and calm your mind.

Meditation or relaxation is integrated with yoga. This helps you to become more aware of the present, with what is happening at the moment, and learn how to accept it without any judgment.

There are studies, which prove that yoga helps in reducing stress and anxiety. The practice also manages your mood and gives you a better sense of well-being. It can also help in combating chronic conditions, such as heart problems, pain, depression and insomnia. It is generally safe for healthy individuals, but it is recommended to begin training with the guidance of a professional.

Precautions are necessary if you are suffering from any of the following health problems. In this case, you have to seek the advice of your doctor before you begin doing any kinds of yoga practices.

Eye problems, such as glaucoma

Pregnancy

Unregulated blood pressure

Herniated disk

Severe osteoporosis

Any health problems where you are at a risk of developing blood clots

Severe problem with balance and posture

If you can't find a qualified trainer near you, make sure that you read and learn more about the practice before you begin with it. No matter what kind of yoga you would want to pursue, it is always necessary to listen to your body. Never push in doing certain poses if you are already in pain. Take it slowly. As your body gets used to the exercises, your flexibility will improve and you will eventually learn how to do the more complicated poses and exercises.

Niyama, the second limb of Yoga, is the counterbalance to Yama, which is described later. Niyama is best understood holistically, but to do so, a momentary decomposition of Niyama is in order. Niyama has to do with the purity of mind, body, and spirit. Purity, as a concept, has been the source of much pain and suffering over the generations. It is the source of the caste system, racial and color supremacy, as well as intolerance. Purity in Yoga, however, is none of these things. Niyama in Yoga is about the total purification of the self at a level that is beyond the tangible and the physical. It is about purity beyond what our manifestations are. Purity is about the clarity of understanding, and to approach the truth.

Niyama is divided into five areas but eventually taken together. It's like making soup – you take individual ingredients, but you bring them all to a boil at the same time. The five are self-purification, being content, determination, study, and surrender.

Self Purification

The idea of self-purification is not limited to keeping one's self clean, hygienic, and neat. The need for purity spans a wider spectrum. It can be as simple as having a shower and keeping yourself superficially clean. But it is also something deeper than that. In Sanskrit, it is called Shaucha. It describes the state of being clean and the act of becoming clean. In Yoga and the various limbs that support it, an act or a conclusion is never the point of the whole thing. The journey, there and back, is just as important. As the axiom goes, it's the journey, not the destination. So too in Yoga, the goals that outline the various limbs and the elements of each limb are about the destination and the journey there.

The same is true about Shaucha. The process of purification when preparing one's self is as much a mental ritual as it is a physical act. As the mind focuses on moving impurities away from the body, it alters the mindset. The new mindset becomes more aware of the impurities that exist and the alteration begins to diffuse into other areas of the person's existence. The architects who developed Yoga found that the intangible mimics the tangible. The reverse is also true. To be able to purify the intangible – some would call soul, it is important to purify the body, but not at the expense of exclusion and derision.

The goal of self-purification is to rid the impurities of the physical existence so that the mind can begin to recognize and remove the intangible impurities within its realm. Cleanliness is indeed next to Godliness, as far as Shaucha is concerned.

Contentment

The second ingredient of Niyama is contentment, Santosha in Sanskrit. The idea of contentment is not about indifference. Contentment in Yoga is about the state of being at peace with one's self and surroundings. It is not designed, intended to depress or discourage ambition and the drive to achieve. Yoga, when properly practiced will provide motivation and clarity in whatever line you choose to direct it.

True contentment only comes when there is clarity. Clarity only manifests when there is purity. Purity only exists when the mind desires it and makes the necessary effort to achieve it. The physical self-purification that was discussed earlier is one example.

To be content requires an understanding of the forces at work and a path of progress that develops an understanding of the nature of things. Yoga is not a superficial art. The mere practice of poses and breathing techniques will show some benefit, but that would only be a tiny tip of a titanic iceberg.

The key, once again is the path to contentment, as much as it is the goal. The path to contentment illuminates the nature of things and reveals what is important and how all else is trivial.

Santosha is about letting go of the past, just as much as it is about letting go of non-essentials. It is the mother of minimalism. When you are content, you can see things for the way they are and it brings you one step closer to enlightenment.

Determination

In Sanskrit, one's determination is known as Tapas. Tapas is not just the willingness and ambition to do something or to see the outcome of the job at hand. Tapas is about the energy that one conjures within, to move with urgency and determination. The key here is that one cannot rush. This grace is not for showmanship, but a deeper concentration of energy. The same physical manifestation of that focused energy is transmitted in the Tapas of Niyama. When one's determination is not rushed, the resulting focus allows the task, or the thought, to be driven to its conclusion. The power of Tapas can then be used during meditation. Tapas is the prerequisite to many areas of one's life, meditation is just one of them.

Develop Tapas by focusing on the matter at hand. Imagine the energy you would have to generate to do something in haste. But don't do it in haste, instead channel that same energy into doing each component task of the objective, one at a time, without pause or distraction. When you practice the Asanas, move from one pose to the next with full determination and without thought or consideration to anything else. Treat your task at work in the same way.

Self-Study

When Shakespeare said, "to thine own self be true," or when the Romans say that "to conquer the world, you must first conquer yourself," they are talking about getting in touch and being with the focal point inside that is the real you. This aspect of Niyama is known as Svadhyaya. Svadhyaya is the ability to get to know who you are and where you fit into the grand scheme of things. The former comes first, the latter comes last. You can't know the grand scheme of things if you don't know who you are. Yoga, however, is not the art of looking inwards. In the grand scheme of things, you need to be able to focus on a point but not at the exclusion of the whole. Self-study is the key to subjecting the values and beliefs you possess to the actions that you manifest. In most cases, they are not aligned until you begin the process of self-study.

It is an art. You merely need to look in on yourself and do it consistently and deliberately. The time for Yoga and Asana should be preceded by the exercises that are contemplative and honest.

Self-Surrender

Ishvara Pranidhana is the term for it in Sanskrit. Self-surrender is about becoming one with the higher power not becoming subservient to something or someone. As a living soul, one person is not subservient to another, we are all part of the same fabric that is Universal. To strive for independence where it is not warranted is like being a single thread woven in the fabric but trying to distinguish yourself from the rest of the fabric by pulling away. It can't be done.

Self-surrender is the ultimate step in the liberation of the true-self in the confines of the physical manifestation. By surrendering the self to the Universe, one is elevated to understand the truth and the power within.

The common thread that runs through the five elements of this limb would make it clear that the Niyama is about jettisoning the baggage and elevating the self. The counterbalance to the Niyama in Yoga is the Yama. We will discuss that in the next chapter. To make Niyama clear, it is worth contrasting the two forces of Yoga. While Niyama is inward-looking and pensive, Yama is outward-looking and active. The two complement each other perfectly to provide a harmonious and seamless existence and form the foundation that is needed in the rest of the limbs of Yoga.

The inward glance and focus are not the same as self-importance. It is about understanding and observation. Just as you would observe the character and personality of someone you just met, you should do the same to yourself.

Often times when you finish with your yoga work out you will find that you feel amazing and there is a good reason for this. It is not simply that you completed your exercise for the day, but it is because yoga works just as well as many medications when it comes to treating any issues you are dealing with.

There is now scientific proof that shows you can heal your own body with the power of the mind. What you believe is what you receive! When you use yoga to relax, the cells in your body release what is known as nitric oxide. Nitric oxide is what dilates the blood vessels in the body and helps to stabilize the immune system. Studies have shown that mind/body methods have worked just as well at treating many problems as the drugs that have been designed to treat them. The only difference is that when you use a mind/body method, you do not suffer from the same side effects as you would if you were taking medication.

We all know that as we age our brains begin to shrink, but studies have shown that those who are practicing yoga on a regular basis actually see the opposite effect, their brains actually continue to grow.

The truth is that yoga, can heal your body, your bind and your soul. It can help regulate your hormones, strengthen your body, help you heal faster from injuries and help to prevent injuries.

There are actually poses that you can use to help heal yourself from the inside out.

Cobra Pose - This pose helps to heal back pain, obesity, menstrual pain and disorders, indigestion and even insomnia.

Begin by lying on your stomach with your belly button sucked in. Place your hands beneath your shoulders and push up gently lifting your torso off of the floor as much as you can while arching your back.

Hold this position for 25 seconds, then lower yourself back down and repeat.

Zen Pose - This pose helps to heal sexual issues, prostate issues, sciatica, joint pain, back pain and indigestion.

Begin by sitting on the floor with your legs bent underneath you and your buttocks on your heals. Make sure that your back is kept straight and you are not hunched over, press your shoulders back and sit up tall. Fold your hands in your lap and focus on your breathing. This pose can be used at any time such as when you are praying or reading, but if you using after eating it will help reduce indigestion.

Head to Knee Bend - This position will help to heal depression, mental illness, anxiety, fatigue, high blood pressure, back problems and joint problems.

Begin by sitting on the floor with both of your legs extended out in front of you straight. Raise your arms up over your head as if you are reaching for the ceiling and then bend forward trying to reach for your toes. If you can reach them, grab them with your fingers and hold the pose for 30 seconds. Release the pose, straightening back up and relax your body. If you are unable to reach your toes, try the position with one leg bent, the sole of your foot pressed against the inside thigh of the opposite leg.

The **downward facing dog** is a pose that we already covered, but it is important to know that it also helps to heal the body from the inside out.

Yoga should be a regular part of your life because it not only heals the body but it also treats mental issues as well. When you use meditation along with yoga, you will find that it helps with many psychological disorders and it is so powerful that it has helped even cancer patients recover. When yoga is unable to treat a disease such as cancer, it helps by strengthening the body as well as the mind.

When you are practicing yoga and meditating, you should not focus on what is wrong with you but instead focus on feeling good. Imagine how your body will feel when it is healed, how your life will be when you are healed. The meditating will help you to manifest your healingwhile the yoga does all of the work. If you know anything about"The Law of Attraction" this will make more sense. If not, I suggest that you look into it, but you should know that what we focus on the most is what we get out of our lives. This applies to our health just as much as any other area of our lives.

Yoga mudra and the five vital elements of the body have a close relationshipe The mudras can be used to balance the five vital elements of the body, which are water, earth, ether, air, and firet Any deficiency or excess of each element can cause a disorder and imbalance in the mind and bodyd The thumb represents fire, the index finger represents air, the middle finger represents ether, the ring finger represents earth, and the little finger represents watere

Mudras for the earth element will include your ring finger

Mudras for the air element will incorporate your index finger

Mudras for the fire element will include your thumb

Mudras for the water element will incorporate your pinky or little finger

Mudras for the ether element will focus on your middle finger

In this post, we are listing the mudras that represent the five elements of the body and the individual benefits it possesses.

Surya Mudra (Mudra of the Sun)

Bend your knees and take a seating position. Keep your neck and back straight. Bend your ring finger and press it with the thumb. Place both your hands on folded knees and put a little pressure in your palm and relax the rest of your hand. Practise this mudra at least twice a day for a minimum of 5 minutes and a maximum of 15 minutes each time.

Surya Mudra is known to sharpen the centre in your thyroid gland. Regular practice of this mudra is known to bring down the cholesterol levels in your body and reducing weight. It also helps to control anxiety pangs and improve the digestion.

Vayu Mudra (Mudra of the Air)

Bend your knees and take a seating position. Keep your neck and back straight. Place your index fingers at the root of your thumbs and press it with thumb. Your index finger should touch the middle fingerPlace your hands at folded knee so that palm is facing up and put a little pressure in your palm and relax the rest of your hand. Practice this mudra for 20-30 minutes every day.

Vayu Mudra is known to prevent all illnesses that occur due to imbalances that are present in the air. It helps control and eliminates the gastric disorders and is known to reduce the intensity of rheumatism, arthritis, joint pains, back aches and sciatica. The Vayu mudra takes a minimum of two months of continuous practice to show better results.

Prithvi Mudra (Mudra of the Earth)

Bend your knees and take a seating position. Keep your neck and back straight. Touch the tip of the ring finger to the tip of the thumb, while stretching out the other three fingers. Place your hands at folded knee so that palm is facing up and put a little pressure on joined tips and relax the rest of your hand. Practice this mudra for 20-30 minutes every day.

Prithvi Mudra is known to reduce all physical weakness and helps to reduce digestive related issues. It helps to clear the toxins from the body thus giving it a healthy glow and keeps your body healthy. This is an excellent mudra for those who want to gain weight.

Varun Mudra (Mudra of the Water)

Bend your knees and take a seating position. Keep your neck and back straight. Touch the tip of the little finger with the tip of thumb, while stretching out the other three fingers. Place your hands at folded knee so that palm is facing up and put a little pressure on joined tips and relax the rest of your hand. Practice this mudra for 20-30 minutes every day.

Varun Mudra is known to balance the water content in your body. Regular practise of this hand mudra prevents muscle shrinkage and is beneficial to keep in control blood as well as urinary related problems.

Akash Mudra (Mudra of the Sky)

Bend your knees and take a seating position. Keep your neck and back straight. Touch the tips of middle finger and thumb and keep other three fingers straight. Keep your hand on your folded knee, remember to keep palm facing upwards. Place your hands at folded knee so that palm is facing up and put a little pressure on joined tips and relax the rest of your hand. Practice this mudra for 20-30 minutes every day.

Akash Mudra is beneficial for people with heart disorders or blood pressure. Regular practise of this mudra is known to strengthen the bones and increase one's spiritual power.

The Table Pose

Can you imagine what a **table** looks like? The table pose is thus called because it's where you make your body into a table. To do this is fairly easy. Sit on your mat and bend your knees so that your feet are completely flat on the floor, holding your arms behind you are shoulder width and placing your hands to support your body onto the floor so that the palms of your hands touch the mat.

Inhale and lift your pelvic area off the ground so that your hands and your feet support you. The danger with newbies to this exercise is that they let the neck get strained. Don't do this. Make sure that you have your head in a comfortable position and let your hands and feet take the strain. As you get used to doing the **table exercise** you will get more efficient at doing it and it will become easier, but do expect this to be a little hard at first. When you feel that you have held the stance for long enough, breathe out and move your butt back onto the mat.

The benefits of the pose are that they help you to keep your tummy in and straighten your spine. They also help you to be able to digest your food more effectively since your stomach muscles will feel stronger. Thus, weight loss becomes a lot easier. The more effective your digestion, the easier it is for your body to process the food that you eat, but remember that you also want to avoid that horrible stuffed up feeling and may find yourself much more comfortable with eating less.

The plank

This is a pose that will take some time to master and is very important because it helps the discipline of your body and your posture. If you approach this in the wrong way, you will find that you are unable to keep your hands flat, so let's get used to feeling the hands flat on the mat in front of you. Kneel down and lean forward, place your hands onto the mat. Put a little weight onto them and make sure that your hands stay flat at all times. The problem happens when you lean too far forward because your hands tend to move a little. Practice keeping them perfectly flat before we go into the plank position. You may wonder why a yoga position is called "plank" but it's basically common sense. You are going to get your body to lie in a straight line like a plank would. Your arms should always be placed at shoulder width apart. The reason that we are emphasizing the placement of the whole hand as opposed to merely your fingers or the sides of your hands is because the hand placed in this way protects the fragility of the wrists and stops you from hurting yourself. Another area that you need to get accustomed to putting weight on is the end of your feet. Holding your hands in the position as above, place the weight of your body onto your outstretched feet. At this stage, you are merely getting accustomed to the places that will take your weight and strengthening them ready for the full pose. This is always advisable when you are new to yoga.

Getting ready for the plank, stand on your mat. Now lean forward and remember to place your hands flat onto the floor. You may have to bend your knees to start off with, but the idea is that you create a downward V with your body so that both sides of the V are straight. The balls of your feet should be on the floor. Now, push your body weight forward so that your body makes that plank. At this stage, your arms will be taking a lot of weight, so make sure your hands stay flat on that mat. Now, let your arms down so that your forearm is resting flat on the mat and take your body down to that level too, straightening it out as you come down to your plank position.

Downward Facing Dog

You may not know it, but during the plank exercise you already did this. This is when your make an upside down V on the mat, keeping the sides of the V straight. You start this position on your knees and lean forward placing your hands flat onto the mat in front of you. I find the best way of doing this is actually to go down from this position so that your forearms are flat on the carpet and walk the legs back until you can bend and touch your forehead onto the mat in front of you. Remember between movements to inhale, move, and exhale, etc. because the breathing matters a lot when you are doing exercises of this nature. When you have been in that position for a moment or two, start to walk your legs forward after lifting your head. Your legs will be balanced on the ball of your foot while your hands will take over the balance at the front as you lift your body into an upside down V.

This is a very popular position and you can then exercise one leg at a time from this position by bending it forward for a moment and then placing it back into position.

These are the basic yoga poses that a beginner should learn and it's important to perfect these before moving on to more complex positions. You may say that this isn't a lot, but that's intentional. It's not about how many positions you can do. It's about using the positions that you learn correctly. These all help to shape up your body but they do a lot more than this.

If you do these poses and make sure that you eat the right foods and drink sufficient water, you will find that the flow of your body will be a lot more comfortable. You not only increase your metabolism, but you also make yourself feel more at peace with the world. At the end of each session, you need to sit calmly and relax and the best exercise that you can do between exercises or movements and finishing your session is to meditate.

Meditation

Close your eyes – concentrate on nothing except your breathing. As you breathe in, don't think of it as just air. It's much more than that. Think of that flow of air as a mass of energy going into and leaving your body. It's pretty hard to think about nothing because we have been taught since childhood to think things through and adult life tends to fill our minds with all kinds of things. What you need to do for the time that you meditate is think of nothing except the breathing.

Breathe in to the count of seven, hold that breath inside you for the count of three and as you breathe out, feel the breath leave your body but also feel the pivoting action of your upper diaphragm. That's correct breathing. As you exhale, count ONE. Then inhale, hold the breath and exhale and count TWO, all the way to ten. If you find that you do get to thinking about anything else at all, start at ONE again and try your best to get as far as ten without thinking about anything else at all. You may think it's easy, but at first you will be interrupted a lot by the thought processes that are going through your head.

Let yourself have a little calm before you go back into your world because that way you benefit from the relaxing effects of yoga to the maximum. You take all the extra inner strength that you gain from yoga back into the world with you and this really is helpful to relieve stress and makes you feel much more in control of your life. In the chapters to follow, I will be telling you where you can get more exercises to help you to develop your yoga experience. For the time being, it's important that you perfect this asanas because they are the most important for beginners. As you learn them, you will feel more confident in your ability and can then tackle more complex poses. Remember not to run before you can walk. There's no hurry and it's better to achieve the positions correctly than to rush forward and try more complex movements.

If you want to use yoga to lose weight then you need to do specific yoga poses. Here are the some of the yoga poses that you should try if you want to lose weight and burn fats:

1. Shoulder Stand

This pose can help if you have thyroid problems. If your thyroid is malfunctioning then you will have weight issues and it will be very challenging for you to lose weight. To do the shoulder stand, you have to:

· Lie down on your yoga mat.

· Inhale and gently pull your upper body up and support your back using your arms and your shoulders.

· Take a few deep breaths while you are in this position.

· Exhale and gently bring your legs down.

Remember that breathing is really crucial when you are doing this pose. If you want to reap the weight loss benefits of this pose then you need to do this at least ten times a day.

2. **Crescent Lunge**

This pose is one of the most powerful fat burning yoga poses that will help you lose weight fast. To do this:

· Kneel on your yoga mat and make sure that your knees are apart.

· Step your left foot forward. You have to make sure that your foot is flexed past your knee. You also have to make sure that your leg is parallel to the floor.

· Inhale and then raise both of your hands above your head.

· Exhale and then raise your back knee.

For best results hold the lunge for ten breaths. Breathing is also crucial to this pose. Remember that you have to pay attention to your breathing and you need to make sure that you are taking long and deep breaths. This pose expands your chest, shoulders and lungs. It strengthens your quadriceps and it improves your concentration and stamina. It also burns a lot of calories.

3. Wind Relieving Pose

This pose burns a lot of calories and it also help burn belly fats.Furthermore, it helps you reduce unnecessary body weight. This pose is mostly used by athletes and dancers to stretch and warm up.

· Lie on your back.

· Take a deep breath. Inhale and extend your arms and your legs.

· Exhale and then bring your knees to your chest. You have to clasp your hands around both needs.

· Hold your left knee and gently release your right leg. Hold this for about 20 long and deep breaths.

· Gently bring your right knee to your chest and wrap your hands around both knees. Hold this pose for about 20 breaths.

· Then gently release your left leg and hold your right knee. You have to hold this pose for 20 long breaths.

· Draw your right knee back to your chest and wrap both hands around your knees.

· Exhale and gently release both legs.

4. **Warrior Pose**

The Warrior pose is one of the most popular yoga poses. This pose will help tone your arms, abdomen and thighs. This pose is often used many times in the Sun Salutation yoga sequence. This yoga sequence is also known for its toning and weight loss benefits.

· Stand straight on your mat and slowly step your right leg about 3.5 feet to the right. Gently turn your torso to the right then rotate both feet to the right.

· Bend your right knee to the right but keep your left leg as it.

· Raise both of your arms above your head and your fingertips must be pointed upward.

· Hold this pose for about twenty breaths.

5. **Triangle Pose**

This pose burns calories and it is a total body workout. It strengthens your abdomen, feet, legs, neck and ankles. This pose also improves your digestive system and it helps relieve stress and anxiety.

· Stand straight and do the mountain pose.

· Then step your feet apart. Keep your legs apart.

· Turn your left foot, knee and leg around by around 90 degrees.

· Turn your right leg by about twenty degrees.

· Raise your both arms to your shoulder level and your palms should be facing down.

· Stretch and turn your body to the left and put your left hand on your left shin. You have to reach as far as you can.

· Raise your right arm. Your palm must face forward.

· Gently look up. Open your chest and look at your right hand.

· Hold this position for twenty deep breaths.

· Go back to the mountain pose or the standing position.

· Do the other side.

It is important to take deep breaths while you are doing the movements. For best results, do this at least ten times a day.

6. **Bow Pose**

The bow pose has many health benefits. It combats respiratory diseases and it also help improve the function of the digestive system. It is also known for it's weight loss benefits. The bow pose help improve the body's metabolism.

· Lie on your yoga mat facing down. Your arms should be on your side.

· Keep your legs apart and slowly bend your knees and grab your ankles.

· Hold this position for ten breaths.

· Release your ankles and repeat this at least ten times daily.

7. Legs Up the Wall

The Viparithakarani pose or "Legs up the wall" pose has a certain rejuvenating effect. This is the reason why it is usually used in restorative yoga. This pose tones your lower abdomen and it calms your mind and body.

· Lie down and slowly raise your legs upward. You have to make sure that your shoulders are on the mat.

· Stay in this position for 10 breaths.

· Gently bring your legs down then relax.

Do this about ten times a day to reap all the benefits.

8. **Bridge Pose**

This pose helps you stimulate your thyroid gland and it helps speed up your metabolism. As a result, you body will burn more fats.

· Lie down on your mat with your arms on your side.

· Keep your legs apart and lift your hips and waist up.

· Hold this pose for ten breaths and then release.

Do this at least five times a day to reap its weight loss benefits. The bridge pose also tones your thighs and muscles. This pose is also perfect for those who have thyroid problems.

9. **Cobra Pose**

The Cobra pose is a very simple yoga pose that strengthens your spine and helps firm your buttocks. It also helps condition your body and it lose weight.

· Lie on your yoga mat facing down. Your hands should be on your side.

· Inhale and slowly lift your chest and back off the mat.

· Hold that position for five breaths and then release.

To reap its optimum benefits do the cobra post at least ten times a day.

10. Twisted Chair Pose

This pose improves your digestion and it helps your blood circulation. It also helps remove those love handles and tone your abdomen.

· Stand straight and do the mountain pose. Make sure that your feet and your legs are together.

· Gently bend your knees and slowly lower down your hips.

· Keep your palms together.

· Gently lower down your hips and your knees and keep your palms together.

· Gently rotate your back. Slowly place your left elbow to your right knee.

· Hold this position for ten breaths.

· Switch to the other side.

For optimum results do this ten times daily.

These poses help condition your body for weight loss. These yoga poses help speed up your metabolism and encourage optimal health .They can even ease body pains. Doing these poses daily will increase your opportunity to have a healthy, well-toned and fit body.

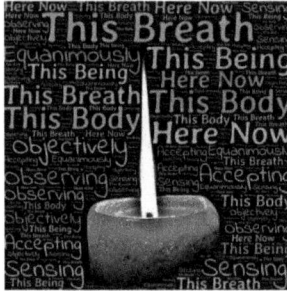

Breathing is an automatic function and often, we seem to be unaware of the importance of breathing correctly. Poor mental or physical breathing habits result in our using only a fraction of our true respiratory capacity. To be able to live a healthy life, fuel is obtained from the foods that we consume. Then, cells within the body start to break down the chemicals in the food reducing them to simple compounds where they release energy, produce water and carbon dioxide. This process is known as metabolism and it requires oxygen to be able to function effectively. As we inhale, the air fills our lungs and as a result, oxygen is absorbed into the bloodstream.

At this same time, carbon dioxide passes from the blood supply into the lungs and is then exhaled. The oxygen rich blood returns to the heart and is pumped around each part of the body. So the air inhaled i.e. oxygen is then transported around the blood by the red blood cells. There is a protein in the body called haemoglobin and this binds with the oxygen enabling it to carry it throughout the body, then the oxygen is released for the cells to use. The brain requires much more oxygen than any of the other organs, it also has a high rate of metabolism. Consider those times when you are unable to think clearly, your instinctive response is to breathe in deeply as this supplies your brain with sufficient oxygen. At those times when you experience mental fog, a lack of concentration or overwhelmed by your emotional state, it often signifies of lack of oxygen.

When you breathe correctly you gain the following benefits:

Greater   concentration
Improved   clarity   of   mind
Greater   ability   to   problem   solve
Improved   emotional   well-being   and
balance   Improved   physical   control
Improved coordination

Understanding   the   importance   of
breathing will enable you to clarify the
relevance to your students as breathing
techniques are a large part of a regular
yoga practice.

There are two sides to the brain, the left
side - often considered the logical and
analytical side and the right side known to
be the creative and emotional side. It is
important that the two sides are balanced
and as with everything in yoga, breathing
exercises help to keep both sides in full
balance.

Left side of the brain

Aggressive Logical
Analytical Rational
Objective
Masculine
Sun
Hot
Yang
Attributes-mathematical and verbal activities

Right side of the brain

Calming
Intuitive
Holistic
Emotional
Feminine
Cool
Moon
Yin
Attributes-spatial and non-verbal activities

When you breathe correctly, the movement exists in three parts. Initially, your diaphragm will cause the abdomen to start expanding therefore, the lower lungs begin to fill up. Then, the intercostal muscles expand the rib cage and oxygen fills the middle part of the lungs. Finally, the collarbone is lifted and air is brought into the top part of the lungs. Unfortunately, many people breathe shallowly and therefore, only the top part of the lungs are used. This shallow breathing can starve much of the body from oxygen, preventing waste products i.e. carbon dioxide from being exhaled.

We've already stated the importance of breathing correctly, but sufficient oxygen levels are vital for the effective functioning of every cell in the body. Without it, the cells are not even unable to metabolise food properly and so vital nutrients will be wasted.

In yoga, the breath is seen as the outward manifestation of prana. This is also known as energy or life force which flows through the body, although, it is actually within the astral body. When visualising prana, it instigates a powerful regenerating force and once controlled, it can be used for self-development purposes and so healing.

Breathingexercises
The breath is seen as a vital link between physical and mental health and pranayama serves to cleanse and to strengthen the physical body, it also helps to clear and calm the mind.
Abdominal breathing

Abdominal breathing should be practised while lying flat on the floor in the corpse pose (Savasana). Practice this breathing technique yourself fully before teaching others. Make sure you focus fully on the breathe and visualise drawing the air into the bottom of the lungs, by extending the diaphragm and noting the abdomen wall as it rises on the inhalation and reduces on the exhalation.

Note: you can check if you are breathing correctly by sitting in a cross legged position or, the Lotus posture and have one hand on your abdomen and the other hand on your rib cage. Inhale slowly and you will feel your abdomen expanding first, followed by the rib cage and then, the oxygen fills the upper chest. As you exhale, the air leaves the lower lungs, then the middle and lastly, the top part of the lungs. You will feel your hands moving as your stomach pulls inwards.

Alternate nostril breathing

This is an excellent breathing technique which can help to reduce stress, provide clarity of mind and even help to eliminate headaches. It strengthens the whole respiratory system. In advanced sessions of alternate nostril breathing, the exhalation will be twice as long as the inhalation and this aids the removal of stale air and any waste products. Initially, practice 5 rounds leading up to 10 rounds per day and keep the in and out breath the same length gradually extending the exhalation.

Close the right nostril with your thumb and then exhale through the left nostril and then inhale to a count of 8. Close the left nostril as well and retain the breath up to a count of 16. This may be difficult to begin with so reduce the length of the hold if necessary i.e. inhale for 8, hold for 8 and exhale for 8. (Build up gradually). Release the right nostril, exhaling for a count of 8. Keep the left nostril closed and then inhale through the right nostril for a count of 8. Once again, close both nostrils and retain the breath up to a count of 16. Release the left nostril and exhale to a count of 8 and this completes one round. Repeat 2 or 3 times. Keep the mind focussed throughout.

Respiratory system cleanse

This is a wonderful breathing exercise that helps to purify the lungs and the nasal passage while eliminating large quantities of carbon dioxide and, any other impurities. Because the exercise calls for a greater intake of oxygen, it helps to renew body tissue, enriching the blood and also helps to massage the stomach, liver and the pancreas.

In a seated posture, contract the abdominal muscles quickly and this causes the diaphragm to rise and force all the air out of the lungs. Then relax the abdomen allowing the air to return gently to the lungs and repeat 20 to 50 times for 3 to 5 rounds.

Normal breathing (lying down) This normal breathing exercise helps bring focus to the importance of breathing correctly and can also help aid relaxation in this lying down posture.

Fold one or two blankets lengthways so that it fits under the lumbar region, the chest and the head and then place another blanket which is folded and can be used as a pillow under the head. Once comfortable, settle down and just focus on the breath. Relax your face, keep your eyes closed. Your gaze should be directed downwards towards the chest, noting the rise and fall of the chest through breathing. Ensure that each breath is smooth and flowing and of similar length for inhalation and exhalation. Focus on the rib cage as it moves and feel the mind starting to become quieter and note the sense of peace. Gradually, the breath becomes slower and deeper.

Do not go to sleep in this posture instead, keep breathing evenly for 5 to 10 minutes. Then remove the support from under the back and lie flat with the blanket under the head only. Bend the legs when ready to finish this exercise, turn over to your side and then, gradually come up with your head down as you do so. Sit quietly and contemplate for a few minutes.

Self-Assessment Tasks

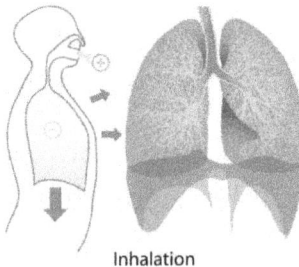

Inhalation

Task:
Practice the various breathing techniques so that the movements become instinctive.

Please note that these self-assessment tasks are to ensure your understanding of the information within each module. As such, do not submit them for review with KEW Training Academy.

CHAPTER 8: HIP RELIEF

One of the most painful places arthritis takes hold is in the hips. If you have arthritis, you know that you need to exercise those sore or inflamed joints, but in the depths of pain that might just not seem possible. There just aren't very many ways to exercise the hip joints comfortably. That's where yoga comes in.

Yoga offers dozens of poses, from beginner to advanced, that can bring a much-needed stretch and some gentle strengthening to the hips. With yoga, you work at your own pace and listen to your body, helping to deliver the relief you need without making your issues worse.

Low Lunge

Sanskrit name: Anjaneyasana

Low lunge delivers a deep stretch to your hips while building core muscle strength to protect your lower back. This pose is also therapeutic for sciatica pain. It does require you to rest on your knee, so if you have arthritis in your knee you'll have to make modifications (such as using a cushion or towel), or choose to skip this pose. You can try starting with High Lunge instead.

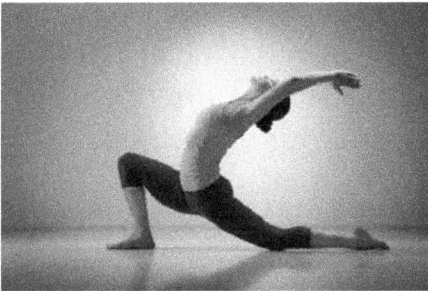

Instructions

Begin in tabletop position. Bring your hands together slightly and move your left foot to the outside of your left hand.

Let your hips draw forward and bring your upper body up, lifting your arms above your head with your hands facing inwards towards each other.

Props

If you suffer from sore or inflamed knees, place a blanket or gel pad beneath your knee when in this posture.

Modifications

If you have trouble balancing in this pose at first, use a chair or sturdy nearby object to help support your body.

High Lunge

Sanskrit name: Utthita Ashwa Sanchalanasana

High Lunge is a good alternative to Low Lunge if you're dealing with knee pain. However, it does require more muscular engagement. Eventually, you want to start building up your muscular strength, because a strong and flexible body helps to prevent the injuries that are so common when you're suffering from arthritis and its friend, osteoporosis.

Like Low Lunge, this pose delivers a deep, cleansing stretch to your hips, lengthening your hip flexors while helping to develop core strength. Core strength is likewise important for preventing low back pain and injury. Because this pose stretches out the front of your body, it's also a good tonic for digestive discomforts.

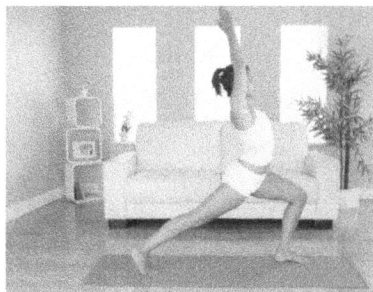

Instructions

Begin in Standing Forward Fold, palms on the floor. On the inhale, bring your left foot through your hands and step your right foot back, resting on the balls of your right foot. Your left foot should be flat against the earth.

Lengthen your torso forward. Rest here with your hands flat against the ground for one breath, and then lift up your torso and sail your arms upwards or rest your hands against your upper thigh.

Strengthen your legs to maintain your balance and breathe deeply to open the chest and front body.

Take a few breaths in your chosen position, and then switch sides. Transition through Downward Facing Dog if you'd like.

Modifications

If the balancing aspect of this pose is too much, lower your back knee to the ground. If that is still too much, place both hands on either side of your front foot.

You can use a nearby object to help you keep your balance.

Warrior I Pose

Sanskrit name: Virabhadrasana I

Warrior I Pose is a foundational yoga posture that you'll find in most yoga classes. Along with brining a stretch to the hips with the slight lunge, and opening the chest, this pose can also bring relief for sciatica pain. For those who want to get deeper into backbends, the Warrior I pose provides a slight bend to the back that can help you prepare for more intense backbends.

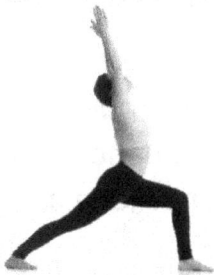

Instructions

Begin in Mountain Pose.

Step your right foot forward about four feet, or as much as is comfortable.

Turn your left foot inward at a 45-degree angle, while your right foot faces forward.

Attempt to square your pelvis as much as possible with the front of the mat. Bend your right knee to a 90-degree angle. Make sure your knee is not collapsing inwards. You can check this by making sure you can see your right big toe on the inside of your knee when you look down.

Lift your arms over your head. Your hands should be facing inwards towards each other.

Breathe deeply to open the chest and create a slight backbend. Hold this posture for 30 seconds, or as long as you need.

Repeat on the other side.

Modifications

If you are dealing with arthritis pain in your shoulders, if may not be comfortable to hold your arms over your head. Instead, place your hands on your hips, hold them in Prayer Hands, or get a deep shoulder stretch with Reverse Prayer Hands, if you can.

Goddess Pose

Sanskrit name: Utkata Konasana

Goddess Pose is one of the best ways to open up your hips and bring a delicious but powerful stretch to your hips and inner thighs. Along with the benefits it delivers to your hips, Goddess Pose also opens your chest and strengthens your core. Although this is a restorative pose, enter with caution as the stretch to the hips and thighs can be as powerful as the goddess this pose was named after!

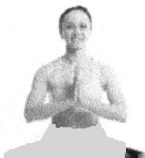

Instructions

Begin standing upright in Mountain Pose.

Step your left foot to the back of the mat, then turn both of your feet facing outwards. You should be facing the side of your mat with your legs spread and your toes pointing to the sides.

Bend your knees to the degree of your comfort until you feel a stretch in your thighs and hips.

Lift your chest and upper body. Ensure that your shoulders are not tense.

Lift your arms above your head for a chest opener or slight backbend.

Breathe here for as long as is comfortable. You may feel some burning and shaking in your thighs. This is normal; however, you should not feel any sharp pain. If you feel sharp pain, exit the pose gently.

Modifications

If you have soreness in your shoulders, hold your hands together against your chest in Prayer Hands. If necessary, you can gently place the palms on the knees for balance, but do not hunch.

Reclining Pigeon Pose

Sanskrit name: Supta Kapotāsana

Pigeon Pose brings a very intense stretch to the hips. Although it's a powerful pose, it might not be right for everyone and has been known to put unnecessary strain on shoulders and knees. Instead, try this modification, Reclining Pigeon Pose or Supine Pigeon Pose, for a slightly more gentle take on the yoga classic.

When you're sitting behind a desk or the wheel of a car all day, you also start to shorten your IT band. Your IT band is the connective tissue that runs from your pelvis down the outside of your leg and down your shin. A tight IT band could be causing unnecessary strain on your hip joints. This pose helps to counteract that.

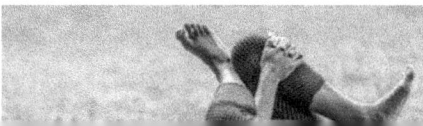

Instructions

Begin on your back with your knees bent.

Cross your right ankle over your left thigh. Cross where ever it feels comfortable, as long as you do not rest your right leg against your left knee.

Lace your fingers behind your left thigh. If you are able to, lift your left leg towards your face. This will deepen the stretch in your hip. Do not lift or put any strain on your neck.

Breathe deeply and hold the pose as long as you need.

Repeat on the other side.

Props

If you do not have the flexibility in your shoulders to reach your leg, you can loop a strap around your thigh and hold on to the strap instead as you gently coax your leg closer to your face.

Modifications

If it's time for a deeper stretch, lace your fingers around your shin instead of the back of your thigh.

Restorative Child's Pose

Sanskrit name: Salamba Balasana

Child's Pose is a key yoga posture that everyone should have in their repertoire. Child's Pose is grounding and relaxing, while granting a space-opening stretch to your hips. One of the best things about Child's Pose is that you can control how much of a stretch you want based on how much you spread your hips. It's also an easy pose to modify.

When we add a cushion or support under the upper body, this makes the pose more restorative, so you can spend more time in the pose without causing any strain. Restorative Child's Pose is a perfect gentle stretch to add in at the end of the day, especially when arthritis pain is keeping you up at night. For this pose you'll need a

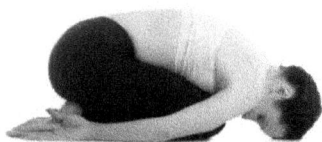

bolster or large pillow.

Instructions

Sit on your heels with the tops of your feet flat against the earth. Spread your knees outwards to your level of comfort.

Drape your body over your thighs, and stretch your arms forward. This would be traditional Child's Pose.

To make this pose restorative, place a bolster, large pillow, blocks, or stack of blankets beneath your torso to support your body.

You can keep your arms stretched forward, or allow them to rest by your side, whichever is most comfortable. Adjust the width of your knees to your desired stretch.

Relax in this pose as long as is needed. Six minutes or more would be appropriate.

Props

This pose calls for a bolster, pillow, blocks, or stack of blankets.

If you have sore knees, you can also place a blanket beneath them.

Happy Baby Pose

Sanskrit name: Ananda Balasana

This pose is a fantastic restorative hip stretch. It also gently massages your lower back and is deeply calming for the central nervous system. That's why this pose is often performed towards the end of a yoga class, to prepare for Corpse Pose. This is a great pose to add at the end of your practice right before bed.

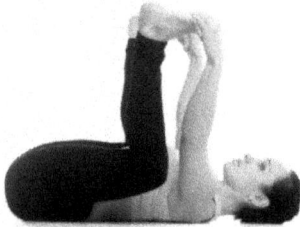

Instructions

Begin by lying on your back on your yoga mat, then bring your knees in towards your chest.

Hold on to the outside of your feet and move your knees towards your armpits.

Straighten your legs to the best of your ability, just enough to deliver a gentle stretch to your hips and shoulders. Your ankles should be stacked above your knees.

If possible, rock back and forth sideways, to give your lower back a stretch and massage.

Props

If you cannot reach your feet, do this pose one leg at a time. Bend one knee towards you and loop a strap around the middle of your foot, then assume the pose with one leg, holding the strap with one hand.

Fire Log Pose

Sanskrit name: Agnistambhasana

This pose is pretty intense for the hips, so you'll want to work your way up to it with more gentle poses, like Child's Pose, first. If you can get to the point where you are doing this pose on a regular basis, you'll practically have new hips. If sciatica pain is also a problem for you, this is one of the best poses for treatment and prevention of that.

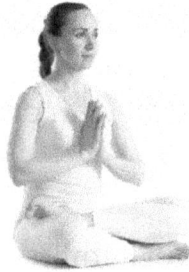

Instructions

Sit on the floor, ideally on a folded blanket, with your knees bent and both feet flat on the floor.

Collapse your right leg so the outside of your leg is on the floor and your foot is in front of your pelvis, as if you were sitting crisscross applesauce.

Stack your left leg on top of the right, with your left foot resting just below your right knee.

Ideally, your legs will lay flush against each other, but realistically, your left knee will probably not reach your right foot. That is perfectly fine, just work on lowering it slowly to the best of your ability.

Breathe in this pose for as long as is needed. It is a restorative pose, so you can take your sweet time here, then switch to the other side.

Modifications

If you'd like to make this pose more intense, straighten your torso, then drape it forward. Inch your hands forward to create length in the spine.

Lizard Pose

Sanskrit name: Utthan Pristhasana

Lizard Pose is an incredibly intense hip stretch, so you don't want to do this pose at the beginning of your practice. Even for experts, this pose is best added in after you've already warmed up the hips and thighs. If you are new to yoga, this is a good pose to have on your radar to work your way up to, but you don't want to try it during your first sessions. However, once you can tackle this pose, it will bring an amazing stretch to the ligaments surrounding your hips.

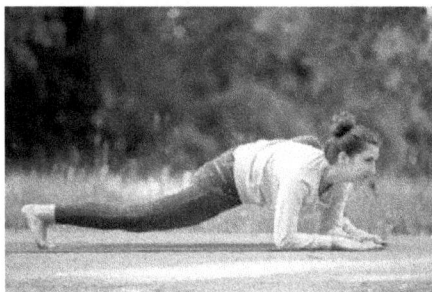

Instructions

Begin in Downward Facing Dog Pose.

Lunge your right leg forward to the outside of your right arm and come down to rest your forearms on the earth. Your foot should be parallel with your elbow.

Do not collapse your neck and chin. Instead, keep your chest open and chin lifted, parallel with the ground.

Keep your back leg lifted to work those leg muscles.

Breathe in the pose for as long as possible, then release into Downward Facing Dog.

Props

If you are not able to reach your forearms to the ground yet, don't worry. Place a block or bolster beneath your arms. You can also stay on your hands.

Modifications

If you have arthritis in your shoulders, this pose might not be ideal. However, you can try lowering your back knee to remove some of the pressure from your shoulders.

CHAPTER 9: POSES FOR MIND CLARITY AND FOCUS

When you are experiencing trouble focusing or you have a bogged down mind yoga is a great way to find some mental clarity and focus. There are many poses that help target these problems, most of them involve the focusing on breathing and how your body moves when you breathe and when you actually execute the move. Here are a few of them.

The Prayer Pose

No, you do not actually pray when you form this pose—while, of course, you often have a similar pose when you do pray. This is "a great way to get in touch with your body and breath" before you go on with your day. It is important to focus on your breathing and to actually breathe deeply through the nose. Improving focus on your breathing will teach you (over time) to focus on other aspects of your life.

How to do it:

Begin by standing straight up with your feet together. You can also have the hip or shoulder width apart; it all depends on which is more comfortable for you.

Now, bring your palms together, in the center of the body. You want to have your hands away from the body, but not too far. You want your hands to be hovering across from the middle of the chest (approximately).

Stay here for a few breaths, making sure that you forget all of you troubles and focus on your own breathing. This pose is all about finding your own peace— whatever that may be for you.

When you do this pose, you can stay in the formation for as long as your legs can hold you up. It really depends on how much time you have, how stressed you are, and how much you need to sort out in your mind. If your mind begins to wander, simply bring it back to the sound of your own breath.

Seated Forward Bend

There are several forward bends in yoga, and they all are known to "quiet the minds and relieve stress". So if there are any big stresses in your life, it may be a good idea to try this move. When you need to improve your concentration - in general or on a certain task - this also may be a good thing to do every day for a few minutes.

Start by sitting on your bottom with your legs extended before you. Make sure your feet are touching.

As you exhale, bend forward and rest your head on your calves (of wherever it falls).

Now, make sure your hands are in the correct position; they should be resting on the floor, palms facing each other and put together.

Stay like this for as long as you feel necessary. When you are in this position, you should breathe deeply.

If you wind it hard or uncomfortable to lay your head completely down on your legs that you do not have to stay like this. If you are new to yoga, you may not be as flexible as you will be later on with practice. So do not feel bad if you cannot stay in this position for long, or if you cannot put your head down.

Along with this, if you feel any sign of light-headedness, it is urged that you stop and slowly lay back and blow your dizziness to go away. Breathe deeply and relax.

The Child's Pose

The child's pose is in the same category as the seated forward bend. By allowing you to focus on your breathing, it promotes mind clarity and concentration. Relieving stress with every breath is the entire purpose of this pose.

Kneel down on a mat (or on the floor, if you do not have a yoga mat). Spread your knees far enough for your whole torso to fit between them.

Now, lean forward, outstretching your hands and exhaling after a nice deep breath in.

Keep your back and shoulders straight as you bend down.

Just like before, with the seated forward bend, you are urged to stop if you feel light-headed or dizzy. It is important to remember, as well, to not go any further than your body can handle. If you cannot bend as far as you see other people bend, ignore that. You will get there if you keep practicing—gaining flexibility and coordination is inevitable when it comes to practicing yoga.

The Mountain Pose

The mountain pose may seem like nothing, and it may seem to not have a purpose, but you'd be surprised at how much this pose can do for your health. There is no need to explain in steps this time, as it is very simple: stand with your hands down at your sides, straightened out. That's it! Doesn't seem very focus oriented, does it?

This pose can even do wonders for your weight, as it promotes toning of the buttocks, abdomen and legs. This pose helps relieve tightness in your body and allows you to destress. It expels dullness and refreshes you.

Standing Forward Bend

As stated earlier, forward bend poses are known to reduce stress, improve focus and mental stability. Here is yet another forward bend pose that you can practice to find clarity in your mind.

You can begin this pose by starting with the mountain pose (explained above).

As you exhale, fold your body straightforward toward the floor and grab your ankles.

Lean your body weight onto the toes. As you lean forward, bring your hands off your ankles and move them to the floor in front of your feet. This is just to support your body weight.

You can hold this pose for four or five breaths for about 30 seconds.

The Camel Pose

The camel pose is one that is said to receive tension and physical stress on the back and neck, as it provides a soft stretch to those areas as well as with the shoulders and arms. The move is said to balance your chakra, helping with your overall being. This can include making you kinder, happier and an overall better person in terms of your behavior and attitude.

On your knees, on a mat or the floor, inhale as you begin to square your shoulders and bend backwards.

Allow your head to call back slightly and reach your hands back towards your ankles.

Rest your hands on the soles of your feet and do not be afraid to apply pressure to them—just don't hurt yourself.

You can hold this pose for as many breaths as you like or you can hold it for 30-60 seconds.

If you have any sort of back problems, this move may not be for you. The literal bending-over-backwards may not be the best for your sore back. Don't worry, though! We have many more poses that you can try out instead.

The Crane Pose

The crane pose is one that requires a lot of focus—and arm strength. Doing this pose takes a lot of practice, knowing how to breathe, and a lot of focusing on your muscles. Before we talk about its benefits and a few warnings, we should look at the pose itself.

When you begin this move, you should start standing; feet shoulder width apart.

Exhale as you bend forward and down to the floor, bending your knees.

Once you've lowered yourself and your knees are parallel with the shoulders, rest your knees close to your underarms and lean forward.

Keep leaning forward until your feet are off the ground and your arms are holding all your weight.

This move makes you focus due to the "nit-picky" places you have to put your knees, and where you find it comfortable. The move is also said to increase your mental strength along with strengthening your forearms. It also increases the flexibility of your spine and is proven to help illuminate or reduce stress and anxiety.

The Dancer's Pose

The dancer's pose is said to improve your digestion and metabolism and can reduce your body weight. It also strengthens the highs, arms, legs, ankles, and chest all while increasing your body's overall flexibility.

At the start of this pose, you should be standing with your feet shoulder width apart. This will ensure that you have better balance.

Now, been your knees up toward your belly and grab your leg right below the knee.

Next, as you inhale, pull your leg behind your back as you lean forward.

Reach your other hand in front of you, palm towards the floor.

You can hold this pose as long as you please or for about 30 to 60 seconds. Your balance may not be the best at first, but if you keep practicing this and moves like it, you should have a good handle on it quickly.

This pose is wonderful for focus, as you need to focus on your balance and the placement of both your hands. This pose is also said to have a good effect of depression, stress and anxiety; virtually swiping it from the mind.

Make sure that you do this pose on both sides—with both legs.

Chapter 10: Breather Exercises And

Meditation

As you can see from the quotation above, yoga helps you to notice more sensations. Thus, it can make you feel sexier, it can make you feel more at peace with the world and it really can work its magic on the way that your body and mind intermingle. In this chapter we look at breathing exercises and meditation because meditation and breathing go hand in hand in yoga, one being a part of the other. If you were asked to sit and think of nothing, your mind would find that quite difficult because in our daily lives, we are expected to think of so many things. It's not normal to switch off. We consider it a failing when we do, though as you will learn, meditation doesn't actually switch off your mind. What it does is allow the subconscious mind to take over. I have used this scenario so many times to describe the subconscious but it's a very relevant one. If you lose something and search for days without finding it, you eventually give up. Then, out of the blue, a thought may cross your mind as to where that item is. You won't know where the thought came from but it solved your problem and you found the missing item. What happens when you rest your mind is that you allow your subconscious mind a little bit of space to perform some pretty spectacular tricks such as in this case. Thus, you can see that switching off isn't a bad thing.

To meditate, you need to sit down. If you can't manage the full Lotus pose, that's alright. Many newcomers to yoga cannot. You may need a small cushion to support you so that you can bend your legs and cross your ankles, but don't worry too much about tucking your legs in like experienced yogis do. Accept your limitations. All things come to he who waits for the appropriate time. One of the most important elements when you try yoga meditation is that your back is perfectly straight. Again, whenever you do anything yoga related – remember the chakras and how important it is for free flowing between them. Remember also to wear comfortable clothes that do not distract you or make you feel their presence.

Be sure that you give yourself the best chance possible to have a successful meditation session. In other words, make sure that you have chosen an area where you are unlikely to be disturbed. If the TV is going in the next room, turn it off. It's going to be hard at first to concentrate on nothing but your breathing, but if you have noises in the background that really will prove a trial. When you are seated in the position suggested, you need to close your eyes. Start by breathing in and placing your hand on your upper abdomen. This is just a trial to ensure that you are breathing correctly. Breathe in and pressing against the upper abdomen feel it pivot as your breathe out. This is important because this pivot means that you are doing it correctly. Practice this for a few moments before you actually start your meditation.

Meditation is where you think of nothing except the breathing. It is easier if you can think of breathing as energy. Feel the energy come into your body as you breathe in, hold the breath for a moment and then breathe out. Use your nose as much as possible because it's more efficient at breathing than your mouth. The problem with mouth breathing is that you have a tendency to swallow air and that really can cause havoc with your digestive system. Get out of the habit because it's really not the most efficient way to breathe.

Starting to Meditate

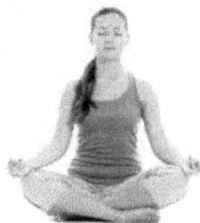

Place your hands onto your knees with your palms facing upward and your thumb and middle finger joined. There is a very good reason for doing this. It stops you from fiddling around with your hands while you are meditating and keeps you grounded in the action that you are taking. Close your eyes. Make sure that your back is straight. Breathe in the energy through the nose and concentrate on that energy entering the body. Hold the breath for a moment. Breathe out through the nose and at the end of the exhale count to one. You use the numbers one through to ten on the exhale and when you reach ten you go back to one again. This is because the numbers should be almost automatic and not something that you need to entangle thoughts in.

Try while you are doing thing to think of nothing but the energy that flows into your body when you inhale and that leaves your body as you exhale. Think of nothing else at all. At first you will find this difficult but you will soon get accustomed to it. Every time that you find your mind wandering, it's a good idea to go back to one again and start again.

Meditation can last up to half an hour though at the beginning, it's good to try for 15 minutes or so.

When you have finished your meditation, put your hands on your lap and relax. Do not move for the time being – carry on breathing consciously through your nose and relax so that you don't jolt your body out of a relaxed state into a state of worrying about what you need to do for the day. Make it a very slow and calm transition to make the most of the meditation process.

What Meditation Does

Meditation frees your mind from thought. It means that you allow your conscious mind to have a break from all of the things that normally invade it. This is important because a stressed person never does this and consequently reaches a point of mental exhaustion. Just as sleep should rest your body, meditation rests your mind and when you have learned to do it effectively, you will find that your levels of concentration are better and that you can achieve more than you usually achieve. Your energy levels are better, and you are more positive in your attitude toward life. It relaxes the mind but it does more than that. It places the body into a position where the chakras can feel the energy flow and thus, you feel fitter.

When you meditate you find peace of mind and that's very valuable in a day and age when everyone is pressured to succeed. In fact, that short amount of time that you put aside for meditation can actually make the rest of your day more efficient because your mind is not cluttered with thoughts. It's rested and ready to take on the challenges of the day.

This makes the perfect time for meditation around the midday point when you need energy for the afternoon, although you should never do it when you have just eaten a meal because you need time for your food to be digested.

As you get more and more experienced at meditation, you will find that you can do it anywhere and that it can help you to up your efficiency and approach difficult situations with a much clearer mindset. Used before a meeting, it can give you more clarity. Used before a difficult family reunion that you have been dreading, it can make you more open to other people and thus more accepting of differences. This helps you to go through your life with a sense of balance and through difficult situations, being able to see that perhaps the situation is equally difficult for others. Your humility comes in useful because it helps you to see the world through other people's eyes and to compromise and find happiness.

CHAPTER 11: WEIGHT LOSS

There is no mystery to weight loss. If you spend more calories than you eat, you will lose weight.

You may need some background information in order to understand how people gain and lose weight.

A calorie is a unit of energy. A dietary calorie is simply 1000 calories. A pound of fat contains approximately 3500 calories.

This means that you will gain 1 pound of fat for every 3500 excess calories that you eat. On the other hand, you will lose 1 pound of fat if you spend 3500 more calories than you eat. The effect is cumulative and it is not time sensitive. There is no "expiration date" on weight gain or weight loss. If you consume 3500 excess calories in one week, you will gain 1 pound of fat at the end of that week. If you expend 3500 calories more than you consume over the course of one week, then you will lose 1 pound of fat. This is true if the timeframe is weeks or months or years.

A three-part plan for weight loss

There are three parts to any successful weight loss plan:

1. Increase the calories you expend

2. Decrease the calories you consume

3. Monitor your progress

Increase the calories you expend

Increasing the calories you expend means being more active. The following examples assume you weigh 275 pounds and that you exert a reasonable effort. The actual number of calories you spend will depend on how much you weigh and how hard you work.

If you do 30 minutes of **Yoga for Fat Guys** five times a week, then you will burn and additional 900 calories per week.

If you add 20 minutes of brisk walking 3 days a week, you will burn an additional 450 calories each week.

If you shoot baskets for 20 minutes three times per week, you will burn an additional 550 calories each week.

Adding these three activities to your weekly routine will burn an additional 1900 calories per week

Decrease the amount of calories you consume

You need to have an effective the eating plan if you are going to lose weight and keep it off. Start by compiling a journal of what you eat, and then look for ways to save calories by substitution or portion reduction.

A typical doughnut contains 300 calories, but a granola bar only has 120 calories. Many fat people routinely eat two doughnuts every day during breakfast. If you make this switch you will "save" 360 calories a day. You will cut 1800 calories each week if you make this switch Monday through Friday.

Change your snacking habits. A candy bar from the vending machine has about 150 calories, but a piece of string cheeses contains only about 50 calories. You will cut 500 calories if you replace one chocolate bar a day with a piece of string cheese five times per week.

You can save a ton of calories by replacing potato chips with fresh fruit. If you have a large grapefruit instead of a bag of chips from a vending machine you will cut about 175 calories. If you make this replacement five times a week, you cut almost 900 calories each week.

Making these dietary changes will cut your caloric intake 3200 calories every week.

Monitor your progress

Your bathroom scale will be a source of constant temptation and frustration. Every day you will step on the scale, expecting huge weight losses. Every day you will get depressed because weight loss is a process that takes time. There is only one way to handle this situation.

Throw away your bathroom scale!

There are three methods to monitor your progress.

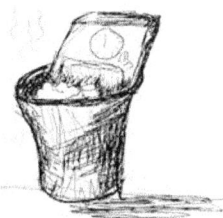

Want to lose weight?
Throw away your bathroom scale!

The Lazy method

The "Button-Down Shirt" method

The "Anal Retentive" method

The Lazy Method

Get a simple heath screening. Have the provider check your weight, blood pressure and heart rate. Do this every six months and keep track of the results.

The "Button-Down Shirt" Method

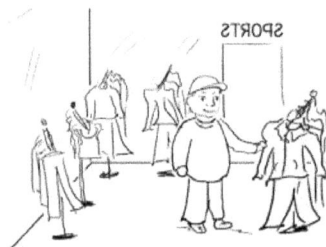

Looking for a good way to check your progress?
Buy some new clothes!

Purchase a shirt that is one size too small for you. Try it on once a week. Eventually, you will be able to button all the buttons and move around without popping a button or bursting a seam. At this point, buy yourself a few new shirts as a reward. You should also purchase another shirt that is one size too small and repeat the process.

The "Anal Retentive" Method

Keep a daily journal of your activities and emotions. Write down the activities that are more difficult because you are fat. Write down the emotional stresses and strains caused by your extra weight. Analyze what's happening to you over time. Look for areas that have improved and identify areas that need improvement.

Exercise versus Diet

The exercise program in **Yoga for Fat Guys** is geared to improving your strength, endurance and flexibility, but it will help you lose weight. You will need to invest six hours each week in the exercise program. You will burn 1900 additional calories per week on this program.

Controlling your diet is far more important to managing your weight than exercise. Controlling your diet is also easier to do, takes less time and costs less money than exercise does. In the example above, three simple dietary substitutions reduced caloric intake by 3200 calories per week.

Dietary substitutions are easy to do; all you have to do is go to a different aisle in the grocery store. Exercise is hard because you have to actually do the exercise.

Dietary substitutions take no time at all, but you have to set time aside to exercise.

You might actually save money by making dietary substitutions, but you might need to spend a few bucks on exercise gear.

This comparison may seem to say "Don't exercise, just diet". I encourage you not to follow that path. Diet and Exercise each have their place in restoring and maintaining your physical health. Dieting is how you lose weight, but exercise makes you strong and fast and durable and makes it possible for you to maintain your weight loss.

CHAPTER 12: EXTENDED TRIANGLE POSE

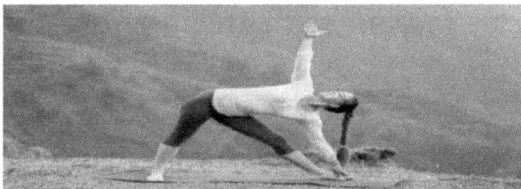

Extended Triangle Pose ('Utthitatrikona') is a more advanced variation on the Mountain Pose, and offers a deep stretch to many leg muscles including the thighs and calves. It can act as a good remedy for mild backache, and offers healthy stimulation to the digestive system.

Start off in Mountain Pose. Exhale, and move your feet so that they are four feet apart. Your arms should be parallel to the floor, out to the side, palms down and with shoulders open wide.

Now you need to adjust your feet. With an exhalation, move your right foot outwards by ninety degrees. Your left foot should be

115

turned in slightly. Your heels should be aligned. Your right knee should be aligned with your right ankle. This is best achieved by making a conscious effort to firm the muscles in your right thigh before turning it   outward.

Now exhale and move your body to the right, over your right leg. You should not bend from the waist, but from the hips – this will help you retain a sense of balance. To retain this position, make an effort to straighten your left leg, keeping the heel pressed   firmly   into   the   floor.

Keep your right hand on your ankle, or use a strategically-placed foam block if you cannot reach down far enough. Extend through your left arm towards the ceiling. Do not strain your neck – keep your head in a soft, neutral position. Inhale and lift your torso out of this position after 45 seconds. As you exit the position, lower your back heel into the mat and push through your outstretched arm towards the sky. Finally, repeat the above

116

instructions with the sides reversed to ensure that both sides of the body are evenly stretched.

Fire Log Pose

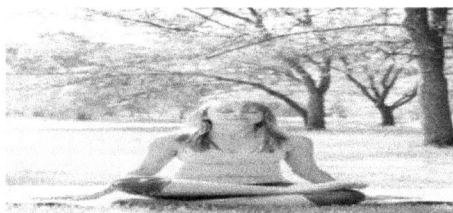

Fire Log Pose ('Agnistambhasana') is often recommended for people who struggle with hip stiffness. It stretches out the muscles in this area, and can be of help for those struggling with sciatic nerve pain.

Roll up your blanket so it is several inches thick. Sit on it, keeping your feet flat on the floor with your knees bent. Sit up straight with your shoulders slightly rolled back. Move your left foot to the outside of your right hip. Position your outer leg down on the mat. Now place your right leg on top of the left. Your right ankle should be positioned outside of your left knee.

Spread your toes. As you exhale, bend your torso forward over your thighs. Place your hands on the floor in front of your shins. Take a deep breath in and notice that your body naturally rises up – when this happens, try and extend the length of spine before folding your torso more deeply over your thighs when you next exhale.
Remain in this pose for 1 minute. Exhale and lift up your torso before slowly uncrossing your legs.

Child's Pose

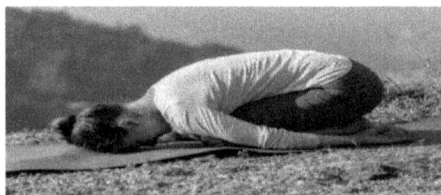

Child's Pose ('Balasana') is a great pose upon which to end a yoga practice, as it allows you to relax and cool down.

Being by kneeling upright on the floor. Press your big toes together. Sitting on your heels, spread your knees so that they are as far apart as your hips. Take a deep breath. As you breathe out, fold your body down onto the mat, between your thighs.

Place your hands on the floor parallel with your torso. Keep your palms facing upwards as you lower your shoulders down towards the mat. Remain in this pose for 30 seconds to several minutes at the end of your practice. To exit the pose, inhale as you lift up your torso.

Cat Pose

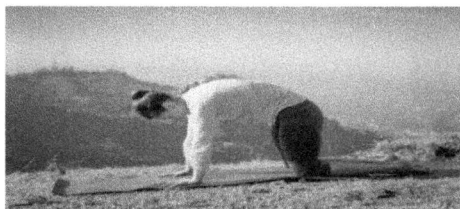

'Marjaryasana,' or the Cat Pose, is a great exercise for strengthening your back and developing spinal flexibility. It stretches muscles in the neck and back and gently stimulates internal organs in the abdomen. Many women find that this pose helps relieve menstrual cramps.

To get into Cat Pose, begin on your hands and knees. Place your hands with palms flat on the floor beneath your shoulders. Keep your knees underneath your hips. Your wrists, elbows and shoulders should all be in a line but not rigid or locked. Do not clench your jaw or neck. Keep your head in a neutral position, eyes looking down at the floor.

Take a deep breath in. As you exhale, curve your spine up towards the sky. As you do this, be sure to keep your knees and shoulders still. As you round your spine, allow your head to drop gently in the direction of the floor

Warrior Pose

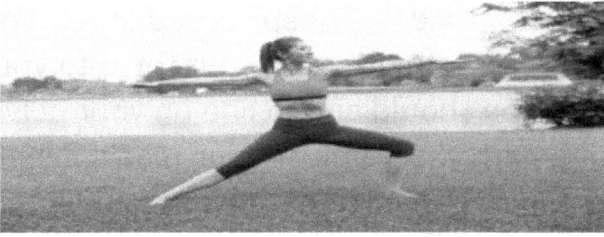

Warrior Pose ('Virabhadrasana') is a commonly-used standing pose that encourages strength, stability and offers a deep spinal stretch. It opens up the shoulders and helps you build stronger leg muscles.

To begin with, get into Mountain Pose. Exhale and arrange your feet four feet apart. Raise your arms so that they are parallel to one another. Stretch through your fingers towards the ceiling. Tense your shoulder blades and imagine drawing the muscles in your back down towards your   tailbone.

Move your left foot 45 degrees to the right, and your right foot out 90 degrees in the same direction. Your heels should be aligned. Take a deep breath. As you release this breath, turn your torso to your right. You should aim to line up your pelvic bone with the front of your mat. Imagine pressing your tailbone down towards the floor, and allow your upper body to arch backwards.

Take a breath. As you exhale, bend your right knee over the ankle. Your shin should now be perpendicular to the floor. Push upwards through your arms and feel your ribcage move upwards. You should feel a stretch through your back leg. Press your palms together. Keep your head in a neutral position.

After 30-60 seconds, exit the pose. Take a breath in, press through your back heel into the mat and straighten out your right knee. Return your feet to their original position then repeat the above directions, reversing the feet as appropriate.

Chapter 13: Some Important Breathing Exercises To Practice At Home

Abdominal Breathing

Sit easily in a cross-legged position on the floor or lying flat on your back in savasana, or corpse pose. Place cushioning under the thighs if you want more support.

Hands should be relaxed at your sides with fingers curling in. Until you master the technique, you may want to place one palm on your stomach to feel the rise and fall of the abdomen.

Relax the mind and body. Breathe in gradually and deeply through the nose. As you inhale, feel the abdomen area fill with air and rise. Keep the chest area still.

As you exhale, notice the abdomen area lower. Repeat this pattern a minimum of ten times to reap the benefits.

Breathing steadily and deeply delivers air to the lower part of your lungs and may significantly enhance inhaling and exhaling capacity.

It calms mind and body, massages internal organs, calms inner thoughts and induces peaceful sleep.

Rib Cage Breathing

Sit comfortably in a cross-legged position on the ground or flat lying on your back in the corpse pose.

Place cushioning under your thighs if you need more support. Place the hands on the sides of your ribcage feeling each rib bone. You want to be able to feel them expanding and contracting.

Inhale slowly from the nostril directly into your rib cage. Avoid pulling the inhale directly into your lungs. Instead, keep it targeted to the area between your ribs between your ribs. Notice how the ribs expand and contract with each inhalation and exhalation.

Repeat the sequence a minimum of ten times in order to calms the mind and the body as well as strengthen the lungs.

Alternate Nostril Breathing (**Viloma & Anuloma**)

Sit comfortably in the cross-legged position on the floor. Keep the backbone and also neck straight but relaxed. Do not lean forward.

Place the support underneath the buttocks or the legs if you'd like more support and stability. Rest your left hand on your left knee.

Lengthen the thumb, finger and pinkie (small finger) of your hand and lower your other two fingers directly into your palm.

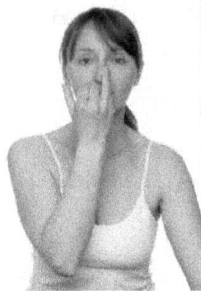

Start by closing your right nostril with your thumb and breathing slowly through your left nostril for a count of eight.

After that, remove your thumb from your right nostril. Press the ring and pinkie fingers against the left nostril sealing it shut from the nasal area. Breathe slowly and deeply through the right nostril for a count of eight.

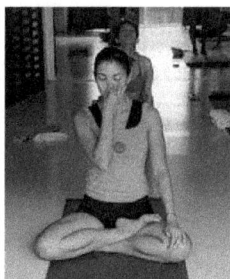

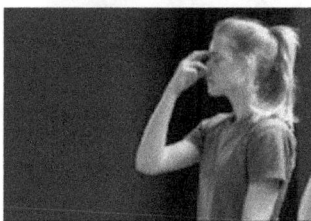

Repeat this series of alternate nostril breathing a minimum of eight times through each nostril. It calms and balances the mind and body, aids in relaxation, increases your ability to focus, and exercises your respiration capabilities.

The Moving Mediation of Yoga

To begin, practice a series of **asanas** which lengthen and strengthen your muscles. Examples might be Mountain Pose or Seated Twist. This series of asanas does not have to be longer than 15 minutes though some people practice a series of asanas for up to 90 minutes.

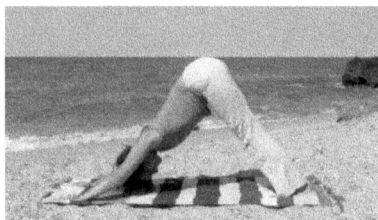

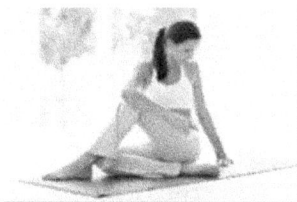

Mountain PoseSeated Twist

Mountain pose assists you in loosening up your muscles as well as gaining control over your brain and intuition.

By gaining control of your thoughts and emotions, you are able to reduce the amount of tension in the body and stress in the mind.

Seated Twist rejuvenates the spine and wrings out toxins in the body. It helps to stabilize the spinal cord and relieves lower back tension.

These poses calm the nerves, bring fresh oxygen to the brain and energize the body, helping to alleviate fatigue.

Additionally they help manage blood pressure levels and assist in restoration in the body and warding off illness by promoting relaxation and rest.

Physically, they improve overall flexibility in the back, sides and hamstrings.

The less strenuous of the poses usually are done at the conclusion of the practice for cooling straight down our bodies and also recover power. Forward bends enhance the blood flow, support digestion and calm the emotions.

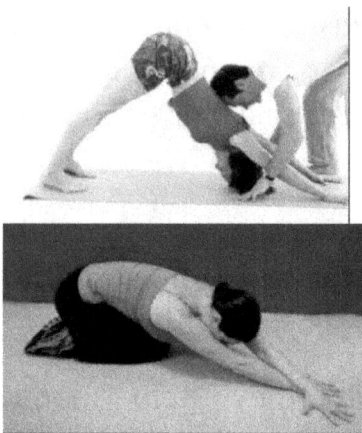

FORWARD BENDTORTOISE POSE

Forward bends and tortoise pose stretch out the lower back and extend the hamstrings. Back bends revitalize and also encourage deep breathing. They open up and energize the body and thoughts.

These poses help to open up the chest area, stimulate the central nervous system, tone the biceps, triceps and shoulder blades, and increase flexibility from the backbone.

Side bends activate the primary organs such as the liver, kidneys, stomach, and spleen. They work to stabilize the body and improve the range of motion in the backbone.

Yogis who engage in these poses advertise overall flexibility within the spine and increased core strength, thus reducing backaches, headaches, and stiffness in the shoulders and neck.

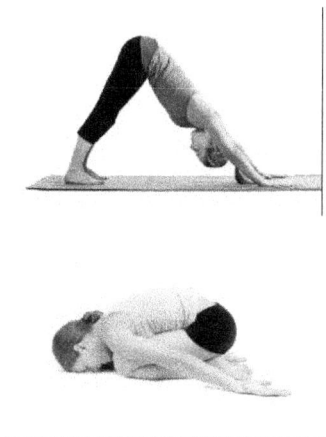

The following series of asanas provides a nicely balanced program inside a compacted **15-minute** of time-period. Choose any combination of asanas and engage in them for 10-12 minutes. End with 5 minutes in savasana, or Corpse pose. This helps you to receive all the benefits of your practice.

FOR FLEXIBLE NECK

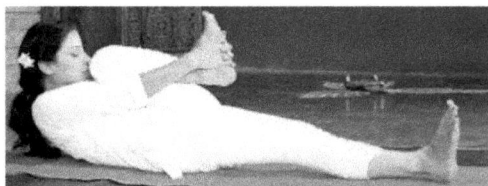

WEIGHT AND FOOD ISSUES

There are several **asanas**, such as the **Sun Salutation** and also the **Fish posture**, that are specific for affecting your endocrine gland. They help to metabolize fat so that it is converted into muscle resulting in a lean, toned appearance.

Sun Salutation Pose

The tendency for people to consume more process foods, refined sugars, fat laden meats and an overabundance of alcohol can wreak havoc on the body. This can manifest in fatigue, mental exhaustion and lack of clarity, headaches, depression and even arthritis.

You have to bear in mind that yoga in and of itself will not heal the body. You also have to make healthy choices like monitoring the quality and quantity of your food, getting adequate rest and sleep, limiting alcohol consumption and exercising self-control.

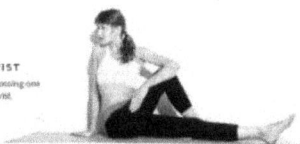

EASY: SPINE TWIST
Unwind your spine by crossing one leg over the other and twist.

The type of yoga you choose to practice may determine the amount of calories you burn during a typical session. Gentle yoga practiced for 30 minutes may result in

100-150 calories burned while more intense yoga like power yoga or Bikram yoga practiced for 90 minutes can burn up to 800-1200 calories per session.

Practicing yoga is effective for slimming down since yoga since the asanas excite the non-active thyroid glands which in turn raise secretions resulting in fat loss.

In pregnancy, yoga advances good health both in the mother and the unborn child. Yoga **asanas** reduce some of the common effects of pregnancy such as excessive weight gain, backache, and depression.

Most women who practice yoga throughout their pregnancies find that their labor is simpler and shorter.

Although several **asanas** need to be adapted during pregnancy, their basic qualities will be suited to women whose bodies are continually changing.

Happy Child Pose is one that provides comfort to women as they start to experience weight gain and pressure in the abdomen.

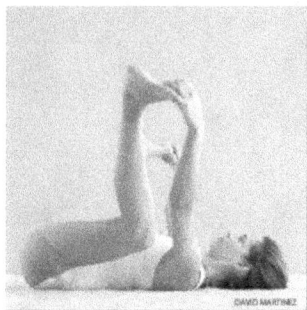

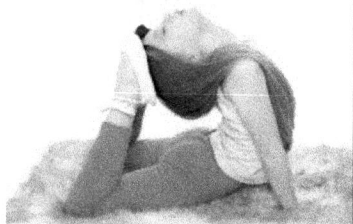

FOR PREGNANT WOMAN

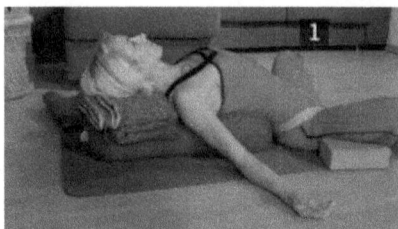

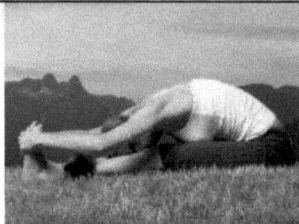

FOR MESTRUAL PAIN RELIEF

Forms of Yoga Poses

Seated poses – Seated poses are beneficial for practicing **Pranayama** and relaxation or deep breathing techniques. Executing seated poses will help enhance your posture and open up your personality.

Standing poses – Position poses are often utilized as warm up for other poses. Standing up poses is helpful regarding strengthening your legs, bettering your stability, and toning your muscles.

Opposite / Reverse poses – Inversions are excellent poses to execute in order to boost the blood circulation, quiet your brain and increase your general health. Inversions are considered to reverse the aging method as well as decrease the effect of gravity on your body.

FLOORBOW

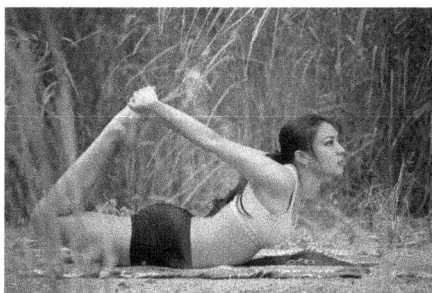

Restorative poses – It is important to consider restorative poses during your yoga practice. They are intended to bring the body back to a balanced state.

Counter poses – Poses like floor bow are intended to exercises the spinal column in the opposite direction of a previous pose and returning it to a neutral position.

Twists – These are great for stretching and improving the spine and the abdominal muscles. Twists improve organ function by providing refreshing blood directly to them.

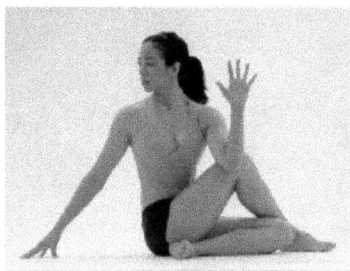

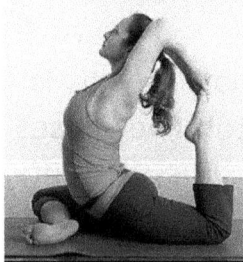

Controlling poses – Controlling poses are great for enhancing your balance and coordination as well as developing your ability to remain still in a pose. Retaining your body in a still pose encourages you to concentrate, quiet your mind and control your thoughts.

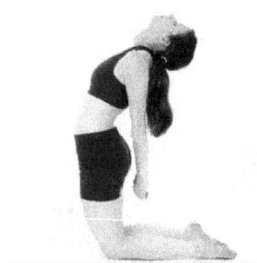

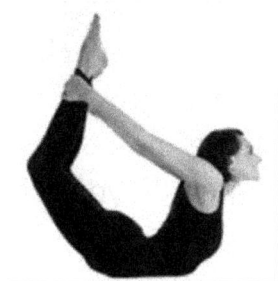

Forward bends – Forward bends extend the entire system, particularly the hamstrings. These are also often thought to calm the brain, comfort your nerves and even release latent hostility. Similar to back bends, forward bends assist in keeping your spinal column robust and supple.

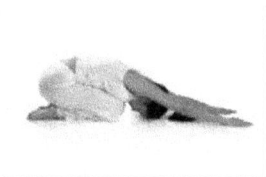

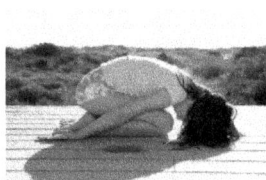

Back bends – Bending backward helps to bring optimal strength to the back and keeps your spine powerful and supple. They serve to open up your chest which, in turn, opens the heart.

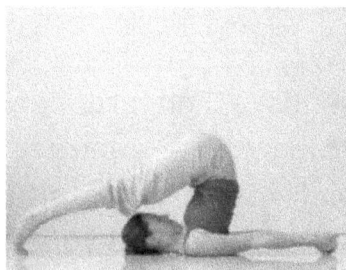

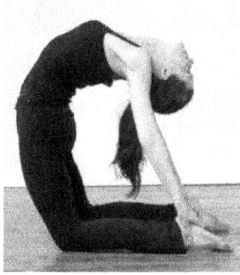

Metabolism can increase so that fat is transformed into muscle and energy. This means that in addition to losing excess body weight, you may gain superior muscle tone resulting in a much smaller, leaner body.

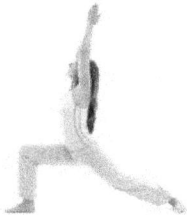

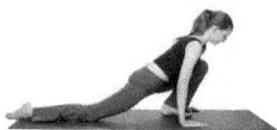

MOON POSE LUNGE POSE

Any pose that relies on placing all of your weight onto a certain muscle group will undoubtedly strengthen that part of the body. Moon pose, Lunge pose, Warrior pose and Triangle pose are perfect postures to lengthen and strengthen the leg muscles.

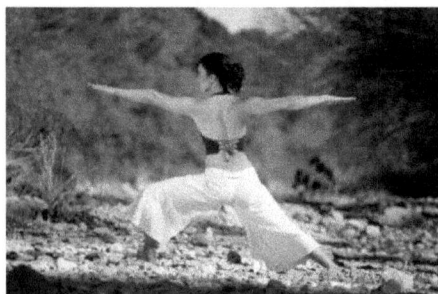

WARRIOR POSE

Cobra, Virasana and Warrior poses are designed to improve cardiovascular health and fitness while improving the condition of your core muscles.

Yoga can be advantageous for everyone's mental health. Because it minimizes anxiousness and stress, yoga can be responsible for causing better health, a more pleasant disposition and a better spirit throughout the day.

COBRA POSE

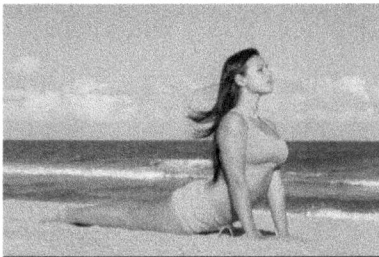

A regular yoga practice assists in boosting antioxidants throughout your body,

143

leading to stronger defense mechanisms and an enhanced capacity speed up the healing process due to illness or injury.

VIRASAN

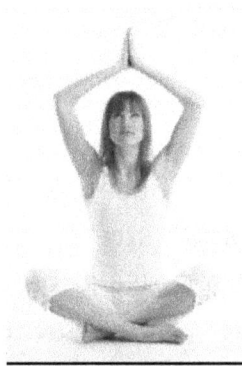

Static Poses are considered to be weight-bearing exercises which increase bone density.

STATIC POSE

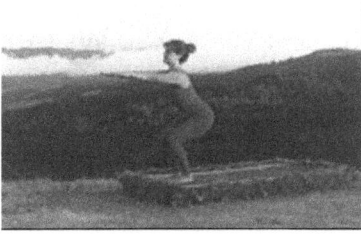

This is particularly advantageous for women who are approaching middle age since yoga might help prevent osteoporosis and damage to bone fragments.

It is well documented that weight-bearing physical exercise strengthens bones so they are less susceptible to weakening with age.

Some poses like Downward Dog, Plank, and Upward Dog require you to simply hold up your own body weight. This type of exercise is great for engaging the core and strengthening the arm muscles.

CHAPTER 14: YOGA AND WEIGHT LOSS

Losing weight is an integration of commitment, disciplined lifestyle and dedication. Yoga helps to lose weight as it's a complete package of good lifestyle and proper healthy eating habits. It is superior to other forms of strenuous exercises and hard-core workouts, as it retains freshness and energy of our system. Ayurveda depicts the importance of reducing the tendency of the body to gain weight rather as opposed to reducing the body weight itself. Yoga is fruitful for gaining as well as reducing weight. Genetics should not be held responsible for being overweight or underweight. Our sedentary lifestyle and unhealthy food habits contribute to weight gain. Power yoga is the most renowned and effective form of weight management. Yoga should be seasoned with determination, dedication and discipline to gain long-lasting results. Pranayam, series of simple activities and positions speeds up the metabolism and hence, aids to reduce the stubborn fat from our adipose tissue. It fosters breathing as a regular and routine phenomenon. Pranayam stimulates the process of slow and steady burning of body fat. Apart from pranayam, there are certain asanas effective in losing weight, the natural way. Yogic jogging and cycling are very reliable for burning the tough fat down the thighs and thus, tones up the body, significantly. Yoga aids to tune with your own body by enhancing self-image and encourages a healthy blissful lifestyle, by providing a sense of well-being. Yoga works by improving the appearance by toning the muscles of our body and improving the posture. Power yoga, is phenomenally popular in health clubs and gyms. There is certain yoga studios dedicated to Power Yoga only. Power Yoga incorporates yoga poses with cardiovascular workouts. It enhances the resting metabolic rate and aids in weight loss. Vinyasa Yoga is extremely popular for weight loss as well.

It is widely known fact that yoga, when done, on regular basis, reduces the level of stress and depresses the production of cortisol (hormone) responsible for tough body fat. Yoga is of restorative nature and connects the person with their own self, by creating self-awareness. It is a great tool for obese people to get the chiseled perfectly toned, attractive physique, they ever carved. Yoga is a natural pain reliever and promotes relaxation and mindfulness. Weight gain is a complex process and is greatly influenced by lifestyle, genetic factors, food addiction and individual will power. Hatha yoga offers profound gifts, apart from its impeccable potential of transforming the body. Yoga works by loosening the muscles of the body that have become stiff a tight by tension, stress and inactivity. Asanas of the Yoga enhance the flexibility, improves the motion of joints and checks the posture that may result in significant weight gain. All styles of yoga sculpt the body by lengthening, strengthen and toning the muscles. Yoga restores the vital energy and reduces sluggishness and weight gain. Yoga is a holistic approach for its physical as well as psychological impacts. Weight gain promotes harsh and tough self-judgment. Yoga reconnects our body and creates a positive and healthy atmosphere for weight loss. Vinayasa or Flow Yoga compels calorie burn at a faster rate as the movements and breath involved in it create a lot of heat. Vinyasa Yoga is a blend of series of Sun Salutation which fosters an increase in heart rate which is critical for weight loss and calories burning. Yoga delivers mental clarity and hence, triggers an obese person on the path of healthy weight loss:

Surya Namaskara (Sun Salutation)

Ardha Chandrasana (Half Moon Pose)

Utkatasana (Chair Pose)

Veerbhradrasana (Warrior Pose)

Uttanasana(Standing Forward Bend)

Badhakonasana (Butterfly Pose)

Ardha Matsyendrasana (Half Spinal Twist)

Setubandhasana(Bridge Pose)

Kumbhakasana (Plank Pose)

Kapal Bhati Pranayam (Alternate Nostril Breathing Technique)

The primary purpose of forward bends is to help keep the spine elastic and not compressed. The exercises under this routine also keep the muscles toned and nervous system revitalized.

Head to knee

In order to achieve the correct head to knee pose, you must relax the body rather than focusing yourself into the position.

How to do it:

Start in a sitting position with your legs straight and arms alongside ears. Inhale as you bring your both arms up. Give your spine a good stretch and bend from the hips.

Draw your upper body as close to your thighs as possible. Hold for 30 seconds. As you release and stretch up, exhale and repeat the pose for 2-3 times.

One Knee Bent

This form of exercise is beneficial for the back muscles. Slouching and hunching over a desk for the whole day weakens and shortens the spinal column. This exercise will help strengthen the back muscles and the proper placement of the spine.

How to do it:

Sit with your legs straight and your right knee bent. Your foot must be flat against your right thigh. Inhale and stretch up your hands as far as you can.

Breathe out and bend your body forward over your straight leg making sure to grasp your toes for some good stretch. Hold to the position for 30 seconds and then repeat with the other leg.

Legs apart

Sit with your legs spread wide apart.

How to do it:

Keep your legs straight, hold your ankles, and relax your neck allowing your head to hang on.

Inhale as you raise your arms above your head and exhale when you stretch forward.

The Butterfly Pose

This particular pose is beneficial for your back posture and in strengthening the leg muscles. Start with a sitting position and avoid hunching your shoulders.

How to do it:

Bend your knees and pull the soles of your feet together. Hold your feet and slowly bring both knees sideward to the floor.

You may also do the half lotus for variation. Sit cross legged keeping your back straight at all times. Your foot must sit on top of the other thigh and the other foot tucked underneath.

The Inclined Plane

You may do this pose after a forward bend. The inclined plane is good in strengthening the arms, shoulders and wrists.

How to do it:

Take on a sitting position with your legs together and feet flexed. Place your hands behind you flat on the floor and your shoulder blades together.

Allow your head to drop back and inhale as you raise your hips. If you are a beginner and you find it hard to raise your hips, you may just sit down with your head back.

Relax on your abdomen

Lie on your front with both hands serving as pillow as you relax one side of your head. Straighten your legs and relax your feet. Now, breathe deeply and do this in between backward bends. This can be an alternative for the corpse position.

CHAPTER 16: HOT YOGA

Defined simply, hot yoga refers to any form of yoga that has done in a heated room. If you are looking to lose weight through it, then you should begin by finding the most compatible form of yoga. For many people, Bikram yoga works the best for this purpose. It comprises of 26 different asanas or poses that are all meant to exercise as well as invigorate your body through and through. It helps in improving circulation as well as toning your muscles.

In this chapter, we'll tackle 10 of the 26 different asanas to help you get started. Remember that as a beginner, you should take things slowly and never overexert. Another thing you must keep in mind would be to become more aware of your breathing. This is important when it comes to Bikram yoga so make sure that you give your breathing a bit of focus as well.

Standing Deep Breathing Pose: Start by pacing each breath. Doing it slowly can help with lung expansion. Next, keep your back straight and do not bend in anyway. Suck your belly in. This can help in straightening your posture. When you exhale, do tilt your head back a bit. Make sure that your shoulders are in line with your hips. You might experience a slight dizziness or a small pinch in your shoulder whilst doing this pose. Don't worry about those as they are normal symptoms if you're doing things right. Hold this posture for about a minute or two before switching.

Half Moon Pose: To begin, stand straight and lock your arms with each other whilst making sure your arm muscles are flexed. Slowly raise your hands upwards, allowing your body to follow the same motion. Feel the stretch and hold this position for a bit before gently bending backwards. Remember, the bend should work its way across the length of your spine and not just in your hip area. The latter might result to an injury so do take your time with this. Once you are comfortable, start bending your hips from left to right. Do this slowly before transitioning to the next posture.

☐**Hands to Feet Pose:** To get into this pose, bend your body forward again, bringing your torso as close to your legs as you can get. Keep your knees straight and locked in while you do this. Make sure that your elbows are placed behind your calves. This might feel like a bit much for a beginner so don't fret if you're unable to do this the first time. With practice, it should get easier and easier. Once you get into the right pose, slowly move your head down towards your shins. In doing this, try to keep your body as straight as possible. Remember to breathe in and out slowly.

☐**Awkward" Pose:** For this pose, you would need to stand tall and straight, with your feet right next to each other. Slowly move your right foot about 6 inches away from your left one. This should create a gap between your knees. Extend your arms in front of you, keeping them flexed and straight. From here, lower your hips gently so your thighs end up parallel with the floor. Hold this position for at least a minute (or more if you can).

Eagle Pose: To get started, stand up straight and keep both your feet close together. Slowly, raise both of your arms and gently hook them together. Your right arm should be under your left one. If you are flexible enough, you can also cross your fingers together to add a bit more stretch to the pose. Next, get in a half-squatting position. Lower yourself enough but do not sit on the floor. Hold the pose for a few seconds before slowly bringing your right leg and placing it over your left one. Your right foot should be touching the calf muscle of your left leg.

Remember, if you can't do it the first time, just stretch enough without hurting yourself. With practice, you'll be able to do this without problem. Bring your shoulders back and push your body upwards from your chest. Hold this pose for about a minute (longer if you can) before going back to a natural position. At this point, switch the positions of your arms and legs.

Tree Pose: Start by choosing a focal point and deepening your every breath. Balance your entire weight on one leg but don't rush this step. Next, use your right hand to hold your right foot up, placing it right in front of your left upper thigh. Make sure that your right foot's sole is facing the ceiling. Tighten your buttocks and straighten your spine.

Make sure that your ribs are drawn in and that your shoulders are moving back instead of forward. Gently open your right hip while slowly working your right knee down then back until both your knees are in a single line. Bring your hands in front of your chest and hold this pose for at least 10 seconds.

Wind Removing Pose: Begin by laying down flat on the floor. Interlace all 10 of your fingers and hold your right leg up, at least 2 inches below your knee. Carefully draw your right knee out and down towards your chest. Slowly pull your right knee to your right shoulder while keeping your elbows close to the body. As you do this, make sure that your shoulders are relaxed and flat against the floor.

Gently tuck your chest in, keeping both legs firmly against the floor. Should your left calf lift, flex your foot. Hold this pose for about 10 seconds, making sure that you breathe deeply as you do so. Repeat the same steps but with the other side of your body. Try hooking your arms beneath your knees if your flexibility has developed. Hold the pose longer with every practice.

☐**Yoga Sit Up Pose:** Start by laying yourself flat on the floor. Pace your breathing and make sure that it is even. Slowly flex your toes upwards and towards the ceiling while gently bringing both of your arms over head. Cross your thumbs. As you sit up, inhale and exhale deeply. Stretch carefully and bend from your hips when you reach for your toes. Don't worry if you have yet to touch your toes. Beginners might need a couple more sessions before they are able to do this.

Hot Yoga Tips for Beginners:

☐For safety, you might want to get a slipless yoga towel, which should help keep you in place while you go through the different poses. You can also get a mat, which should make sitting or standing on the floor much more comfortable. There aren't many different accessories that you'll need besides the basic. Don't forget to bring a bottle of water too! You will need this to stay hydrated during the session.

☐When picking out clothes, do avoid baggy articles of clothing or anything that's made out of cotton. You will want to have a full range of movement and anything that's too baggy might be too uncomfortable for you once you start sweating. Cotton actually traps sweat and would be very uncomfortable, not to mention, quite unhygienic after a while. Tighter and quick drying yoga clothes are your best bet for this purpose.

☐If this is your first time trying out hot yoga, do be aware of the fact that the room you will be working out in can get really hot. For first timers, the change in temperature is often overwhelming but if you give it enough time, you should get used to it soon enough. First, find a comfortable spot in the room and try to sit still for a few minutes. You will feel uncomfortable at first but allow your body to adjust. Try to avoid walking around too much, as this can make you sweat before you really need to. Should you feel dizzy, try and stick around for a few minutes more to see if the feeling would go away. If it persists, however, do speak to your instructor about it.

☐You already know the fact that hot yoga is among the most vigorous varieties of the practice, but did you know that its pace could vary from one instructor to the next. Do not expect slow, meditative sessions though. For the most part, instructors would get you going by using fast-paced, rhythmic music. There are those who don't use music at all. However, it all comes down to your preferences and what will allow you to focus better when exercising.

☐Breathe! The importance of breathing cannot be emphasized often enough. There have been cases wherein people began feeling nauseous or faint during a session just because they were not breathing properly. Should this happen to you, take a break and rehydrate yourself. Catch your breath and make sure your heart rate has calmed down before you even return to doing any poses. Pushing yourself despite your body's signals can lead to injuries or to a fainting spell.

☐Lastly, if you are driving home or taking public transportation after class, make sure that you take a few moments to re-connect and relax before going out of the building. You will feel light-headed, a kind of floating sensation, which is normal especially for beginners. So take five, gather yourself before anything else.

Chapter 17: Yoga Exercises For Beginners

These are exercises that you can perform after you have been through a warm up session and feel safe with. However, don't push yourself too hard. The idea is not to strain yourself but to be totally aware during your sessions of your body movements and your inner feelings. It's about being self-aware and knowing your bodily needs, rather than about fast action packed exercise. You won't lose weight faster, you won't help yourself to center and you won't carry on if you push yourself too hard.

The Lotus position for beginners

You have probably heard of the Lotus position but when you Google it to see what it is, you may be a little discouraged.

Don't be. As a beginner, you are not expected to take the full Lotus Position

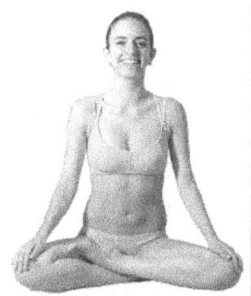

stance.

See how the legs are tucked right up in this image. You won't manage this at first, so simply bend your knees and cross your feet in front of you, rather than trying to bend them to this extent. You will learn to do this with time, though beginners should never try to push themselves into this position until they are ready for it and find that it comes fairly naturally.

Centering your focus

Before you start to do your exercises, you need to center your focus on your inner self. For this exercise, place your hands on your knees with your hand shaped into the format shown in the image. This concentrates you on the yoga if you then close your eyes and concentrate on your inner self. It's worthwhile doing this for a few minutes just to prepare the body for the exercises which follow because it centers you upon the purpose of yoga. Meditation does this but this position helps you to incorporate an element of meditation into your yoga session.

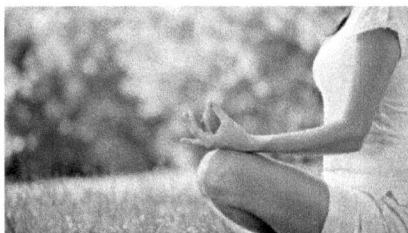

An alternative to this is praying hands which can be performed as per the image below.

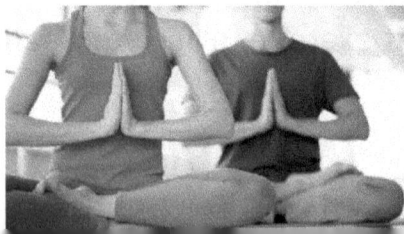

If you have problems with concentrating focus inwardly on your hands and try not to let any thoughts interrupt the process.

Neck Rolls

These help to release stress in the neck area. Keeping the Lotus position, move your head to the right slowly until you can't move it further. Don't push yourself beyond your limits. Then move the head to the left until there is no more movement possible. Move the head to the center. Repeat this four times. Then look upward as far as you can and move the head down so that your chin touches your chest or as near as you can get without straining yourself. Move the head back to the normal position. Repeat three times.

Shoulder rolls

Shoulder rolls are beneficial because your shoulders take on a lot of strain and this helps to loosen them. Sitting in the Lotus position pull your shoulders as high as they will go and then move them forward and around, finishing in the starting position. Relax. Repeat this exercise four times.

Leg exercises

For this exercise, sit in the position shown in the illustration:

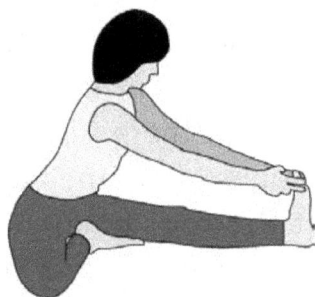

Start in the seated position, tucking your right foot in as far as you can to your left leg. Don't force it. Then, lean forward and try to touch your toes. Again, don't strain yourself and take your time with the exercise. Then move back to the seated position with your hands by your side. Repeat the exercise five times for each leg.

Chapter 18: Pranayama – Weight Loss
Breathing Exercises

It's hard to imagine how a simple series of breathing exercises can literally melt away unwanted fat, but it does...and most effectively too! Pranayama is a Sanskrit word that means 'extension of the **prana** or breath' or 'extension of the life force'. This one word is composed of two Sanskrit words – **prana** (life force or vital energy) and **'ayama'** (to **extend or draw out** as opposed to restrain or control).

Pranayama promotes harmony of body, mind and soul; it calms frazzled nerves and rejuvenates tired cells. It is one of the most efficient of practices and has proved invaluable in the treatment of various diseases, including obesity.

You might possibly be wondering how achieving a state of calm can promote weight loss, but when you think how stress triggers off unhealthy food habits and food choices, you will understand how a balanced state of mind can help you achieve a healthy, weight-controlled body.

Pranayama must be practiced outdoors or at least in an open doorway. If there are trees and plants all around, it will elevate your experience. For even better results, practice Pranayama under a Neem tree, as the curative properties of the leaves enter the air and find a passage into your lungs.

Pranayama is an important part of Yoga because **prana** is the very essence of life. To purify this energy, draw it out, and allow it to fill your lungs through the most efficient of breathing techniques, is to lengthen your life span by enhancing your health.

Remember that you must not eat any heavy meal for at least two hours before you begin your Yoga session.

Sit on your Yoga mat in Padmasana, or Lotus Position, which is with your legs crossed so that your right foot is placed on your left thigh and your left foot is placed on your right thigh. This position automatically straightens your spine, but you must adjust your position so that your spine is as erect as it can be. Look straight ahead and do not allow yourself to slouch. Close your eyes and focus on the tip of your nose.

Begin to breathe deeply, focusing on the passage of air into your nostrils and out. When you have done this for a minute, you can begin the first Pranayama exercise.

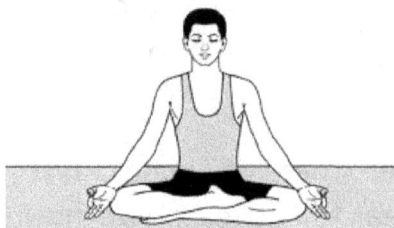

Bhastrika Pranayama

Bhastrika in Sanskrit means 'bellow'; and the breathing technique is akin to the blowing of the bellows.

You may practice Bhastrika fast or slow, but heart patients and people with lung problems need to be cautious, and should either practice this Pranayama very slowly, or seek to practice it under the guidance of a Yoga teacher.

The regular practice of Bhastrika allows your body to imbibe copious quantities of oxygen, as the breathing technique involved is highly efficient.

Stay seated in Padmasana with your hands resting on your knees.Breathe in through your nose forcefully. Feel your diaphragm expand and move down, forcing your abdomen out, and expanding your chest. Ensure that your lungs have expanded to their full capacity. Hold your breath for a fraction of second and breathe out through your nostrils forcefully. Feel your collar bone drop, your chest deflate, and your abdomen sucked in as you exhale.

Repeat Bhastrika for two minutes initially and work your way up to longer durations. Ensure that both inhalations and exhalations are of the same length.

The advantages of practicing Bhastrika Pranayama

The ultimate breathing technique for energy and power

Raises metabolic function at the cellular level to increase fat burn and promote natural, healthy weight loss

Purifies your body by eliminating toxins and waste

Builds lung capacity and helps clear and strengthen the respiratory system

Improves the efficiency of the digestive system

Kapalbhati Pranayama

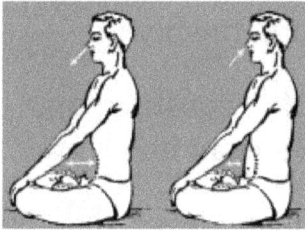

Seated in Padmasana, your right hand on your right knee and your left hand on your left knee, with your eyes closed, take a deep breath. Fill your stomach with air and then exhale with such force that your stomach goes quite deep into your abdominal cavity. As the air is emitted from your nose, imagine all the negative energy in your body being expelled. Repeat this multiple times, resting in between if you need to. Do not inhale and exhale too fast. Be slow and deliberate. The exhaling should be forceful rather than hurried.

The benefits of Kapalbhati Pranayama:

Reduction of belly fat

Elimination of toxins from the body

Reduction of fat in the body

Elimination of constipation, acidity, diabetes and even hair loss

Reduced creatinine levels and improved kidney function

Note: Avoid this Pranayama if you are pregnant. If you are a heart patient, do not exhale too forcefully. If you have High Blood Pressure, then practice this Pranayama very slowly. Women may avoid Pranayama practice during a period, though there are no significant contraindications if you choose to go ahead and practice Pranayama while menstruating.

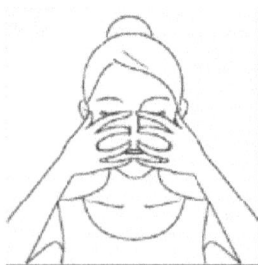

Bhramari Pranayama

Bhramari means 'Bee'. This particular Pranayama exercise is ideal for releasing feelings of anger and frustration, and practicing it promotes mental stability and calmness.

When you are calm and stable, your body is not stressed and therefore does not generate cravings for unhealthy food or inordinate quantities of food. The result is weight control.

Seated in the Padmasana pose, press down gently on your tragi with both your thumbs. Place the index fingers of each hand on your forehead and cover your eyes with the rest of your fingers. Now inhale deeply and deliberately. With your mouth closed, exhale with a humming noise. As you repeat this exercise, you will feel refreshed with positive energy as your body releases impurities.

Advantages of practicing Bhramari Pranayama:

Reduces hypertension

Cures sinus problems

Relieves tension, anger and anxiety

Controls High Blood Pressure

Note: Do not practice Bhramari Pranayama if you have ear problems. Do so only after these problems are treated.

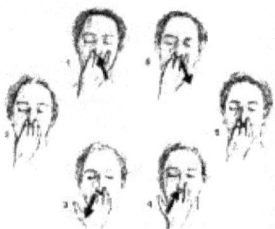

Anulom Vilom Pranayama

The regular practice of Anulom Vilom Pranayama re-energizes your body and relieves stress and anxiety. You should ideally practice it early in the morning on an empty stomach, with fresh air surrounding you.

The amazing benefits of Anulom Vilom Pranayama:

Considered to be very effective for weight loss

It is effective in dealing with conditions like constipation, flatulence and obesity

Improves blood circulation

Calms the mind and reinforces the nervous system

Prevents diabetes and eliminates heart related problems

Promotes glowing skin

Improves lung function

Removes blockages in arteries

Improves concentration

Note: It is best to practice Anulom Vilom Pranayama under the guidance of a Yoga teacher. Pregnant women should never strain while practicing Pranayama. Never practice Anulom Vilom Pranayama soon after a meal. You must have a gap of at least four to five hours between your last meal and the time you practice Pranayama.

Seated in the Padmasana poseyou close your right nostril with your right thumb and inhale through your left nostril. Now close your left nostril with both middle and ring finger, hold your breath for a moment, and then remove your thumb from your right nostril and exhale. Remember to inhale and exhale for ten slow counts each time, and only take air into your lungs and not your abdomen.Continue for at least ten minutes.

Chapter 19: The Koan Of Yoga

EMOTION

The first detriment is emotion. The big, brawny, swaggering bull of emotion. The immediate goal of yoga is the conquest of emotion.

People are ruled by emotion. We don't realize it. It's hard to see most of the time. But we can see it in others. There it's often clear: the green-eyed monster of jealousy, the red-eyed bull of anger and all of their cousins stand out starkly; but in ourselves emotion is so disguised, so invisible.

Emotion is one of nature's tricks to get us to do what nature in general, or nature in the big picture, or nature as the evolutionary force wants us to do. We get **mad**. We feel **hurt**. We want **revenge**. We want to **kick butt**. We are sad. We are happy. We love. We feel exhilaration. We feel **power**.

All of these and many other feelings are the glandular, the neurochemical imperatives that also society through the evolutionary mechanism uses on us to get us to do what it wants us to do. Wave the flag. Hurrah for our side. Love the leader, hate the enemy.

In general, in the long run, for the general animal good, an emotion serves a useful purpose. Fight or flight to save our lives. But if we see someone else with a member of the opposite sex whom we think is in some sense "ours," oh, what horrors will transpire! We perceive a threat to our security or to the expression of our precious genes. To make sure that we aren't substituted for, the evolutionary mechanism makes us cry out: **Get jealous!** And the more ferociously the better. Never mind that we might kill ourselves in the process. Never mind that our precious genes are not really so precious. Never mind that the "damage" may already be done. We have to get mad and we have to risk life and limb and fill ourselves with hate and revenge.

Because that's what the gross, blind and fairly crude evolutionary mechanism requires we feel. It hasn't yet evolved a better technique for controlling us. Having built us a step at a time, through an incredibly long period of trial and error, it has arrived at this rather drastic way of doing things, and only after countless further horrible, painful and totally catastrophic errors will it arrive at the best, most efficient, most beautiful and most spiritual way of doing things—and then only in the very long run. Maybe.

Thus it is said we are "becoming." We are places along the way to becoming. And the games and the techniques and the little hustles of the evolutionary process that are currently being expressed and tried out in us, guinea pigs that we are, will some day cease. And we will have **become**.

WHO AM I?

Many thousands of years ago before we humans were completely human, before we had civilized ourselves, domesticated the pig and the cow, before we learned farming or how to keep track of the seasons, we became aware of the forces within ourselves and without and we asked why are they there? And the answer was always silence or just the wind that blew across the plain. And even though we had no answer, we asked the more profound question: Who am I?

This is not a question an animal asks itself.

And some thousands of years ago the answer came out of the fertile valley of the Indus River and has echoed down through the millennia in the Vedas to us: Thou art that.

This answer when it came to the West in the 19th century seemed to the rationalist mind to be non-responsive, maybe even flippant.

Thou art that.

Ah, but what is "that"? For the mystic, "that" is everything there is, the entire cosmos and everything in time and space forever forward and backward, eternal and beyond mere being and this illusory existence; in short "that" is **Brahman**.

But the first people who formulated this "answer" and tested it in the fire of their souls and found it true, could only express it by analogy—**thou art that** like a drop of water is the ocean.

And beyond this metaphor, the rational mind could not grasp and cannot grasp. And even though there's been an industrial revolution and political ones by the score, and even though the atom has been split and a computer can (or will soon) do a trillion calculations a second— even though the confidence of modernism has given way to a deeply skeptical postmodernism, the answer hasn't changed.

We are still that.

WHY IS THERE ANYTHING AT ALL?

Or we might ask the profound question: **Why is there anything at all?**

This too is not so much a question as a discovery. Why indeed is there anything at all? Why isn't there nothing? Just asking such a question makes one wide-eyed with wonder and initiates one into the inexpressible.

These are both philosophical and spiritual questions. They are profound inquiries into the psychological nature of people and into our "predicament," as it is sometimes called. What is sought isn't mere knowledge but liberation. We want to know, and we want to be set free.

The Bible says the truth shall set us free, but it can't be any textbook truth, any you-told-me and I-accept-it truth. It's got to be an I-lived-it truth.

Yoga is primarily an attitude, a way of looking at ourselves, at the world we live in, and at that something that is greater than we are. Yoga is a way of seeing, a way of knowing and a way of acting. But yoga is above all else a practice. It is something we do.

The yoga that can be learned from books is only the partial yoga. The yoga that is talked about is only a bit of the whole yoga. The yoga that is practiced by others is their yoga and can never be ours. The yoga that is ours is everything we are, everything we do, everything we believe.

Let us end our beginning with the koan of yoga, this fervent "Who am I?"

THE ZEN KOAN

In the Rinzai school of Zen Buddhism the aspirant is given a koan by the master, typically a paradoxical or cryptic query that defies explanation. What was your face before your parents were born? and What is the sound of one hand clapping? are famous examples. After a while the aspirant is given a more sophisticated koan. One of my favorites has the master point to a girl crossing the street and ask, "Is that the older or the younger sister?" Perhaps the most universal is simply Mu? meaning what is Mu? where the word "Mu" signifies nothing.

The idea is to give the student a question he cannot answer with his logical mind—and let him wrestle with it until he reaches a meditative state of mind, and through that meditation after long and earnest practice achieves an enlightenment. Some of the answers that have been found acceptable typically involve a rejection of the question, a non-verbal response (such as sticking out one's tongue), a seemingly irrelevant response (such as "I draw water; I cook rice") or even Bah! The beginning of wisdom comes when the student realizes he truly doesn't know.

In a similar vein we have the story of Zen master Hui-k'o, who would become the Second Patriarch, asking the First Patriarch Bodhidharma to pacify his mind.

Bodhidharma replied, "Bring your mind here before me, and I will pacify it."

"But when I seek my own mind," said Hui-k'o, "I cannot find it."

"There!" snapped Bodhidharma, "I have pacified your mind!"

(I got this story from **The Way of Zen** (1957), a masterwork of erudition and insight by Alan Watts.)

The point was to get Hui-k'o out of the shallows of his verbal thinking and into the depths of actual experience. Let's not be verbal or pretentious. Let's be modest and, above all, concrete.

 "NOT THIS, NOT THIS!"

The famous Vedic answer to "Who am I?"—"Not this, not this!"—evolved into and is the same thing as "Thou art that." But this answer isn't the same thing as saying "I am God" because, for one thing, as the question is asked we and God are separate. The religious tradition that grew out of yoga calls the soul of a human being (the essence of us that is eternal) the **Atman**, and the Supreme Divine Consciousness is named **Brahman**. The goal of yoga is the union of the two.

Thou art that.

Neither the question who am I? nor the answer thou art that can be understood with the ordinary mind To work on our koan, we must nonetheless try some answers.

PEELING THE ONION

We might give our name, Jane Williams. But we are more than our name. We might give our occupation. But we are more than our occupation. We might then try to sum up in words what we are, like a child giving a complete address: "Jane Williams, 123 Main Street, Houston, Texas, U.S.A., Western Hemisphere, Earth, Solar System, Milky Way Galaxy..." We might say that we are the atoms of our body, organized in a particular way. We might say that we are human beings with a certain complexion and body type, with a certain education, living in a certain way. We might even say that we believe certain things and don't believe others. After we have said all these things we have not gotten any closer to answering our koan.

"Who am I?" allows us to peel away the layers of identification like onion rings until we come to the place where there is nothing left—and still we won't know who we are.

Conclusion

Try out a foot stretch or a foot strengthener. See how much better your feet can be.And, remember that it does take a little time for your feet to feel better. Your feet won't get stronger and become more flexible overnight. It probably took years for your feet to get to this uncomfortable stage, and it will take a little time to reverse this process. Be consistent and stick with it. I've had so many people come back to me and say that these exercises have helped their feet. I know that they can be helpful for you as well. Give them a try, and feel better, sooner.

Finally, on a personal note, I've had my own bouts with plantar fasciitis. I've used the toe stretches and the toe lifts to help my own feet feel better. It doesn't take a lot of time out of my day, but it does take consistency. I know that when I've been neglecting my feet and that they start to hurt, then it's time for me to stretch and strengthen my feet. I'm like everyone else. I get busy and forget about all that my feet do for me. However, having a little plantar fasciitis in my feet is a great reminder for me to take time for my own self-care.

There's no better time than right now for you to join me in taking better care of your feet! Grab a yoga block or a massage ball and begin today.